Clinical drawings for your patients

Rheumatology
Second edition

by John D Isaacs PhD MRCP
Professor of Clinical Rheumatology,
University of Newcastle-Upon-Tyne, UK

Illustrated by Dee McLean, MeDee Art, London, UK

Series Editor: J Richard Smith MD MRCOG
Consultant Gynaecologist, Chelsea and
Westminster Hospital, London, UK,
and Honorary Consultant Gynaecologist,
Royal Brompton Hospital, London, UK

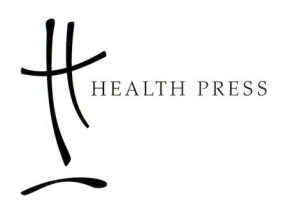

HEALTH PRESS

Oxford

Patient Pictures – Rheumatology
First published 1995
Second edition 1998
Reprinted 2002

© 1998 Health Press Limited
Elizabeth House, Queen Street,
Abingdon, Oxford, UK OX14 3JR

Patient Pictures is a trademark of Health Press Limited.
All rights reserved. No part of this publication may be reproduced, stored in a retrieval system, or transmitted in any form or by any means, electronic, mechanical, photocopying (except under the terms of a recognized photocopying licensing scheme), recording or otherwise, without express permission of the publisher.

The publisher and the author have made every effort to ensure the accuracy of this book, but cannot accept responsibility for any errors or omissions.

A CIP catalogue record for this title is available from the British Library.

ISBN 1-899541-16-0

The author wishes to thank his colleagues at Addenbrooke's NHS Trust who helped in the preparation of the first edition of this book.

Dee McLean thanks Jane Fallows for her help with the illustrations.

Typeset by Impressions Design & DTP
Bicester, UK

Printed by Arkle Print, Northampton, UK

Reproduction authorization

The purchaser of this *Patient Pictures* series title is hereby authorized to reproduce by photocopy only, any part of the pictorial and textual material contained in this work for non-profit, educational, or patient education use. Photocopying for these purposes only is welcomed and free from further permission requirements from the publisher and free from any fee.

The reproduction of any material from this publication outside the guidelines above is strictly prohibited without the permission in writing of the publisher and is subject to minimum charges laid down by the Publishers Licensing Society Limited or its nominees.

Sarah Redston

Publisher, Health Press Limited,
Oxford

Author's Preface

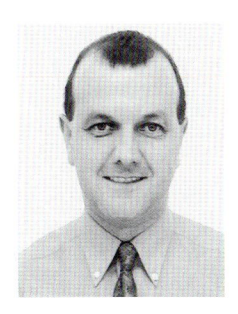

This book is for healthcare professionals to use with their patients. It aims to help you to prepare patients for their first visit to the rheumatologist and the treatments they may receive. Rheumatologists work as part of a multidisciplinary team with physiotherapists, occupational therapists and other healthcare workers. This team treats a variety of conditions, from sports injuries to osteoporosis and arthritis. Although some of these conditions are amenable to simple treatment such as a soft tissue injection, others may involve protracted care shared among the team.

It can be very daunting and confusing for a patient attending the rheumatology clinic for the first time, particularly with a polyarthritis or multisystem disorder. What are the roles of the different medical staff? Why are there so many different forms of treatment? Some patients may wish to know how tennis elbow is dealt with, and how the injection is given. Others may be bewildered by the extensive examination they receive when all they have is painful hands; and who are the physiotherapist and occupational therapist? What are splints for?

Hopefully these words and pictures will remove some of the anxieties and maximize the benefit your patients receive from their first and subsequent visits to the rheumatology clinic.

John D Isaacs PhD MRCP
Professor of Clinical Rheumatology,
University of Newcastle-Upon-Tyne, UK

Arthritis, the joints and surrounding tissues

- Joints are structures where bones meet. Healthy joints allow easy movement between the bones.

- Ligaments are tough white bands of tissue that hold the bones together at a joint. Muscles are the tissues that provide the power to move the joints. Tendons attach the muscle to the bone. Cartilage is a tough, slippery tissue that coats the ends of the bones and prevents the actual bones rubbing together.

- Arthritis is inflammation of a joint, and leads to pain, stiffness and sometimes deformity. Although many joints may be affected at the same time, some forms of arthritis affect only one joint. Gout, for example, commonly affects just one big toe.

- 'Wear and tear' arthritis or osteoarthritis usually affects the joints that hold most of our weight, which are the hips, knees and back.

- Rheumatoid arthritis – another common form of arthritis – often starts in the small joints of the hands and feet, but can affect any joint, including the neck and jaw.

- Less common forms of arthritis are associated with skin conditions such as psoriasis, or bowel disorders such as colitis. Others can follow infections, particularly viral infections, and gut infections that cause diarrhoea and food poisoning.

- Different types of arthritis need different treatments.

Joints of the body

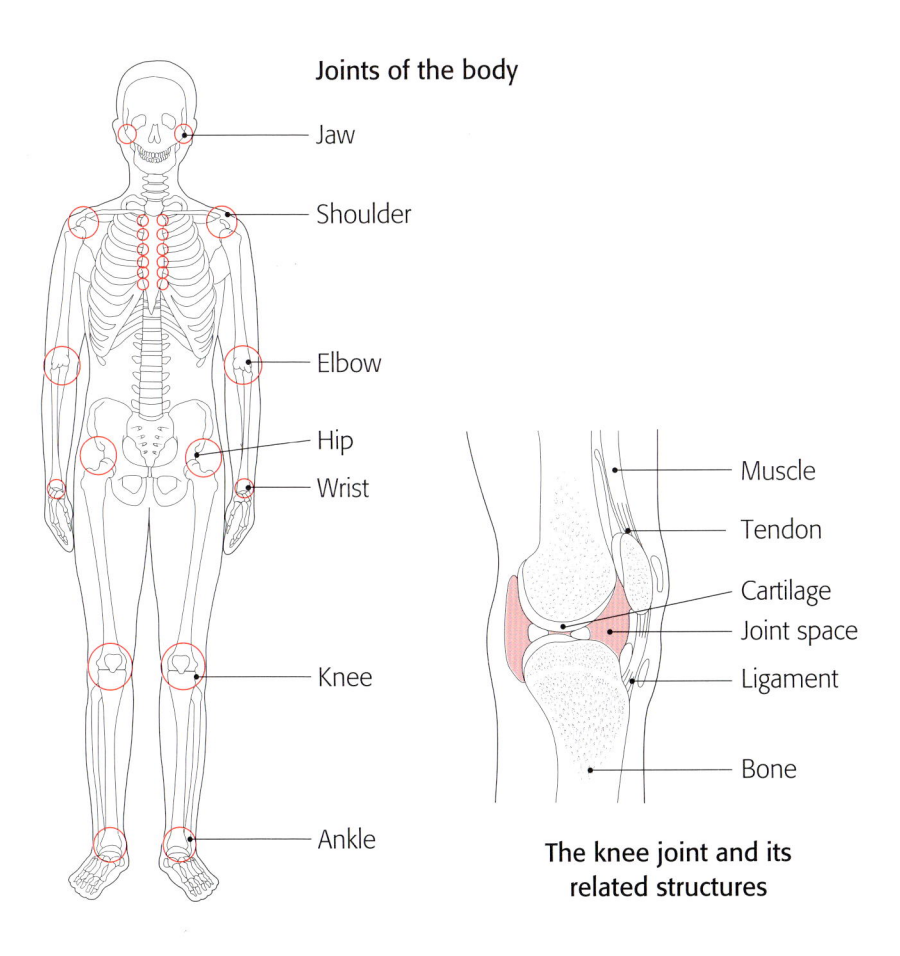

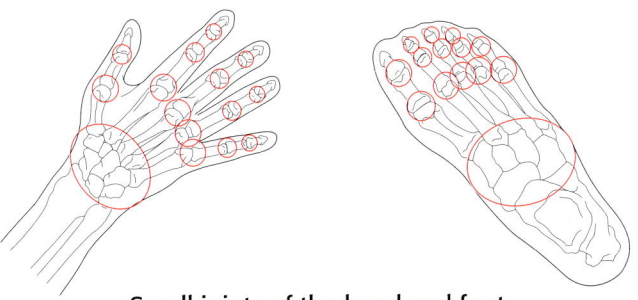

- Jaw
- Shoulder
- Elbow
- Hip
- Wrist
- Knee
- Ankle

The knee joint and its related structures

- Muscle
- Tendon
- Cartilage
- Joint space
- Ligament
- Bone

Small joints of the hand and foot

Arthritis and other body organs

- Some arthritic diseases can affect other organs as well as your joints. Examples of the organs that may be involved are the eyes, skin, heart, lungs, kidneys and nerves.

- An important aim of your visit to the rheumatologist is to find out if any other parts of your body are affected. This will help the doctor to decide what is the best treatment for you.

- So, for example, you may be asked questions about rashes, chest or stomach pains, and pins-and-needles. As well as examining your joints, the doctor may listen to your heart and lungs with a stethoscope, examine your eyes, or feel the area around your stomach.

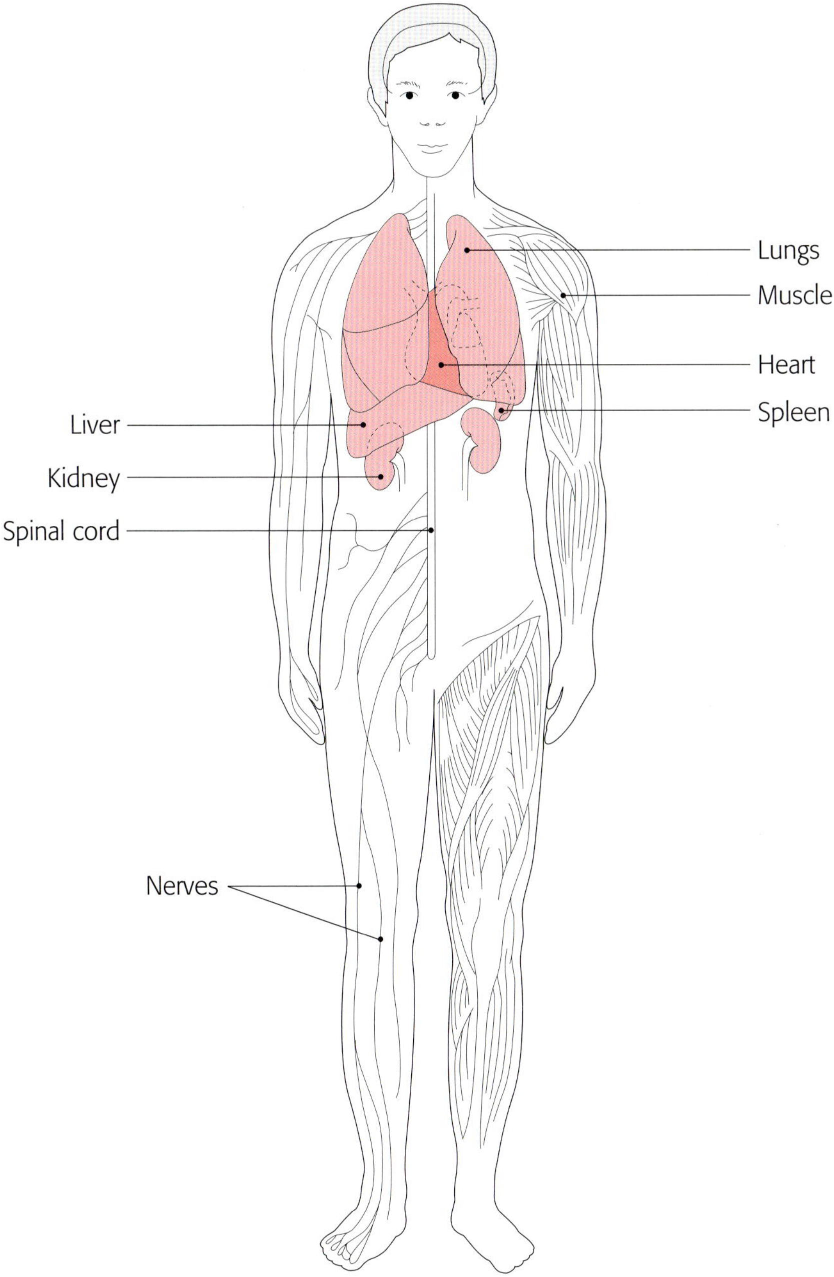
Lungs
Muscle
Heart
Spleen
Liver
Kidney
Spinal cord
Nerves

Osteoarthritis

- Rheumatism is a general term used to describe pain in bones, muscles and joints. Arthritis is a disorder of the joints themselves, and causes pain, stiffness and sometimes deformity.

- The two main kinds of arthritis are osteoarthritis, or 'wear-and-tear' arthritis, and rheumatoid arthritis, which is an inflammatory arthritis.

- In osteoarthritis, the joint cartilage (the tough, slippery tissue that usually coats the ends of the bones within the joint) gradually becomes worn down until the bones rub against one another. This type of 'wear-and-tear' arthritis is more common in older people. Pain tends to be worse after activity, and at the end of the day.

- Painkillers are commonly prescribed for 'wear-and-tear' arthritis. The mildest – paracetamol – may be enough to relieve the pain. Stronger painkillers often contain codeine and may cause constipation. In some patients, non-steroidal anti-inflammatory drugs (or NSAIDs) are also used to give pain relief.

- Changes in lifestyle can dramatically relieve the symptoms of osteoarthritis. Losing weight, taking regular exercise and wearing sensible shoes are all helpful.

- If your pain is not adequately relieved by painkillers and lifestyle changes, you may be referred to an orthopaedic surgeon. He or she will consider whether a joint replacement is likely to help you, and will discuss this with you.

Side view of a normal knee

- Knee cap
- Cartilage
- Joint space
- Bone

Osteoarthritis
'wear-and-tear' of the joint

The cartilage wears down and the bones rub together

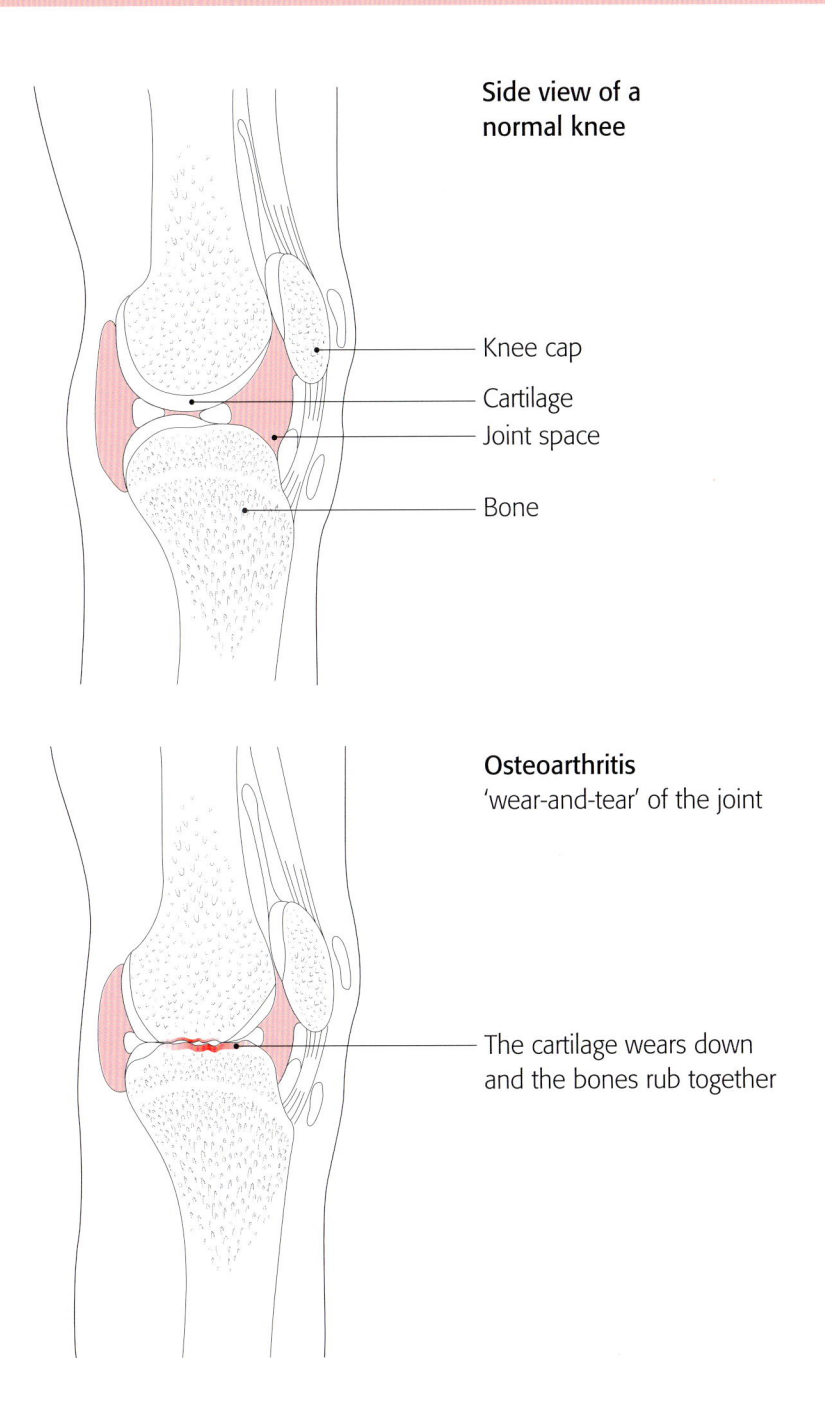

© Health Press Limited

Rheumatoid arthritis

- Rheumatism is a general term used to describe pain in bones, muscles and joints. Arthritis is a disorder of the joints themselves, and causes pain, stiffness and sometimes deformity.

- In rheumatoid arthritis, the tissues within and around the joints become inflamed, and the joints themselves become filled with fluid and white blood cells. The joints become red, hot, swollen, painful and stiff. The pain and stiffness are usually worse after periods of immobility (for example, first thing in the morning).

- If rheumatoid arthritis is not controlled well enough, the inflammation leads to thinning of the bones and damage to the joints, tendons and ligaments.

- Many drugs are available to treat rheumatoid arthritis. Some, such as steroids and non-steroidal anti-inflammatory drugs, control the inflammation. Others slow down the damage to the bones, tendons and ligaments. As well as prescribing the appropriate medicine for you, your doctor may refer you to a physiotherapist, occupational therapist or other specialist to assist in your treatment.

- Occasionally, patients with rheumatoid arthritis are referred to an orthopaedic surgeon. Surgery may be needed to remove severely inflamed tissue from a joint, or in some cases, to replace a badly damaged joint. The surgeon can also repair tendons that have become damaged as a result of inflammation, especially in the hand.

Side view of a normal knee

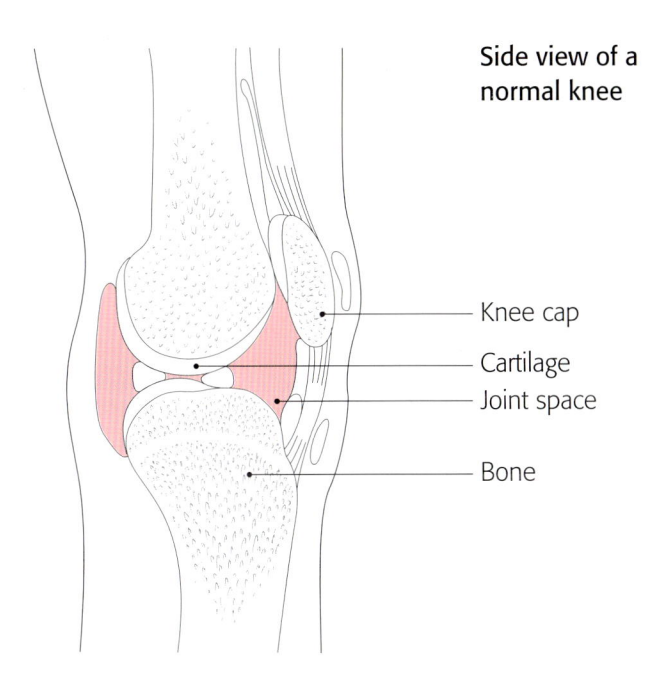

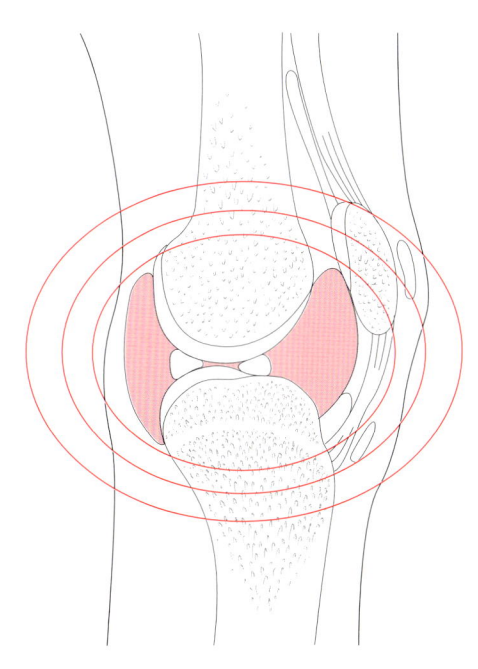

- Knee cap
- Cartilage
- Joint space
- Bone

Rheumatoid arthritis
inflammation of the joint

The tissues around the knee become inflamed and the joint becomes swollen with fluid and white blood cells

Gout

- Gout occurs when crystals of a chemical called uric acid collect in your joints. This causes severe pain, redness and swelling. The big toe is usually affected, but your other joints may also hurt. Bursae, which are pockets of fluid lying just beneath the skin near to the joints, may also be affected.

- If your gout is severe, the gouty crystals may occur in other places, such as under the skin or in tendons. They may leak through the skin, showing as a chalky white substance.

- When gout first happens, your doctor may take a sample of fluid from the painful joint with a syringe. This is important because the symptoms of gout are similar to those of a joint infection, which would need antibiotics.

- You will usually be given an anti-inflammatory drug to help relieve the symptoms of your gout, or a drug called colchicine.

- If you have several attacks, you may be given a drug to try to stop the crystals from forming. Allopurinol is the most common one used. Probenecid and sulphinpyrazone are others. If you are started on these drugs you must not stop taking them suddenly. If you do, you may have a severe attack of gout.

- Certain foods can make gout worse, so you may be referred to a dietician as part of your treatment.

Gout

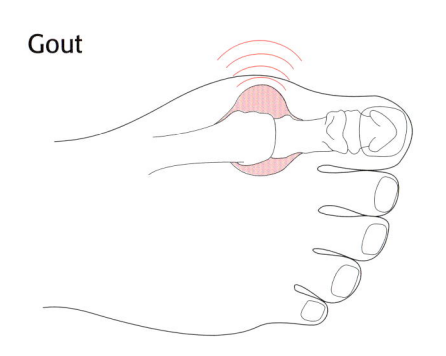

Classical gout affecting the big toe

Gout can also affect other joints, and bursae

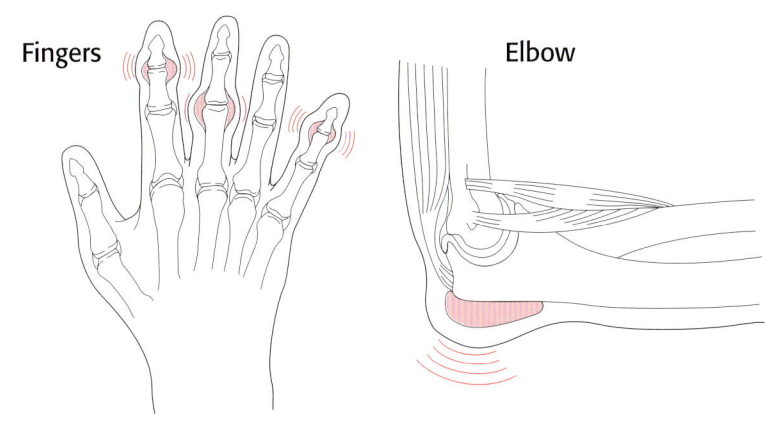

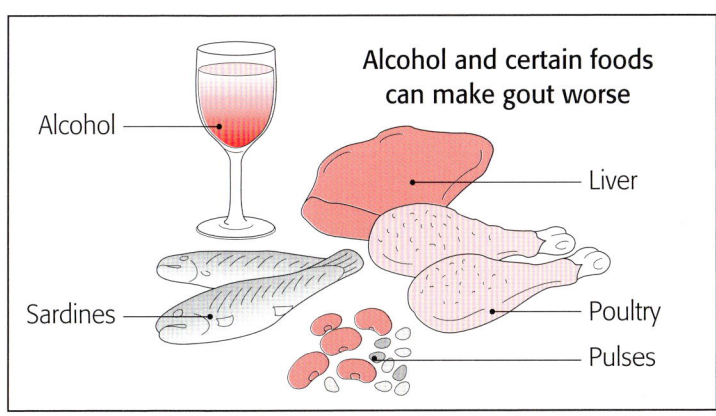

Fingers

Elbow

Alcohol and certain foods can make gout worse

- Alcohol
- Sardines
- Liver
- Poultry
- Pulses

Monitoring arthritis

- Different measurements are needed to monitor your arthritis and its response to treatment. This is especially important for rheumatoid arthritis.

- How far you can move a joint is a very important measurement. A small loss of movement resulting from inflammation or damage may be corrected with physiotherapy and occupational therapy, so it is important that this is discovered early on.

- When a joint becomes inflamed, the muscles moving that joint may waste, or shrink and weaken. Simply measuring muscle bulk or size using a tape measure is a good indicator of muscle wasting and its response to treatment with physiotherapy.

- Various measurements can also show the mobility of your spine, which is particularly important in inflammatory back disease.

- The change in the number of painful or swollen joints with time is a sign of response to treatment, as is the length of time that your joints remain stiff in the morning.

- Your 'functional ability' may also be measured. You may be asked to fill in simple questionnaires, with assistance from a doctor or nurse, about how you cope with daily activities, your level of pain, and general well being.

- Simple blood tests are a guide to the level of activity of your arthritis. They also show up side-effects of drugs you may be prescribed.

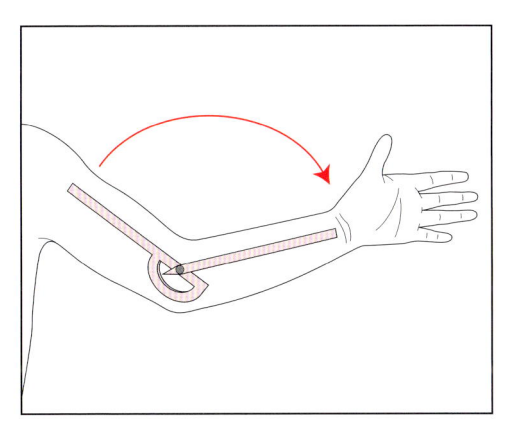

Measuring how far you can straighten your elbow

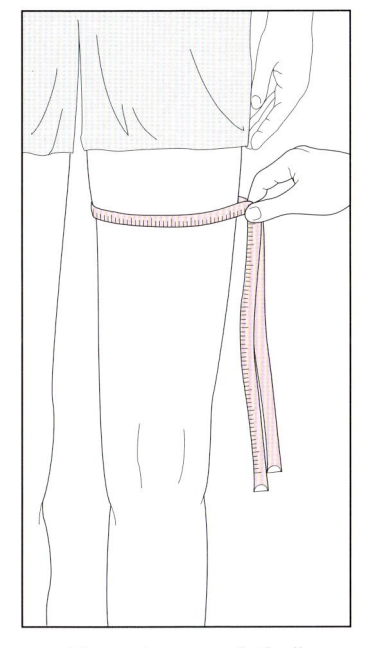

Measuring muscle bulk

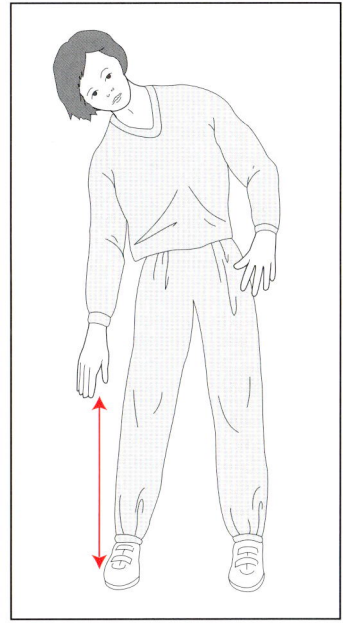

Measuring finger-to-floor distance gives a measure of spine mobility

X-rays and other imaging investigations

- Imaging is like taking a picture of the inside of your body. It helps the doctor to diagnose your problem.

- Taking X-rays is one way of imaging your bones and joints. This is usually enough to distinguish between arthritic conditions, because inflammation and 'wear-and-tear' look different on the X-ray.

- A CT scan takes several X-ray pictures at different points throughout the joint, rather like slicing through a loaf of bread. It shows the joint in more detail than a standard X-ray.

- An MRI scan is similar to a CT scan, but is particularly good at highlighting damage to the ligaments, tendons and muscles. CT and MRI scanning are commonly used to investigate back pain and sciatica when an operation is being considered.

- Having a CT or MRI scan involves lying still for up to 30 minutes within a scanner. Although some patients find being in the scanner a bit claustrophobic, it is not at all painful.

- Ultrasound scans can detect inflammation within a joint or damage to the surrounding tendons and muscles. A jelly-like substance is put onto the skin, and the ultrasound scanner is moved over the area.

- A bone scan highlights areas of abnormal bone and joint inflammation. It is sometimes used when inflammation is suspected, but X-rays are normal.

MRI scanner

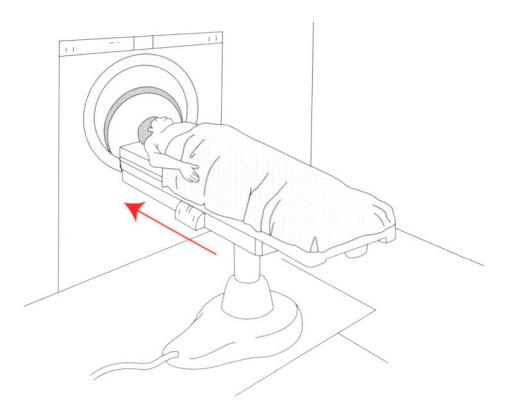

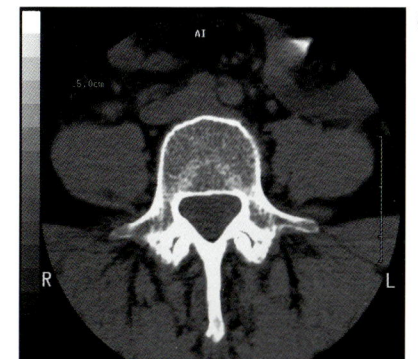

CT scan

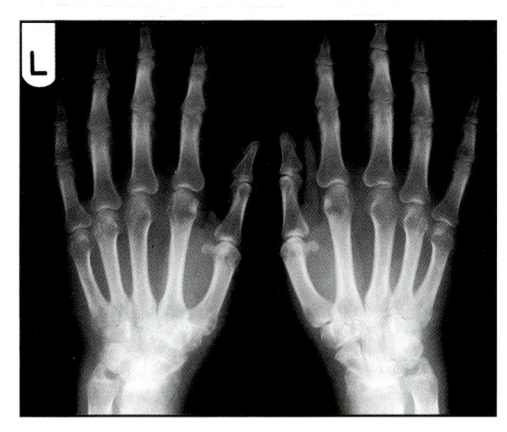

X-ray

Joint aspiration and injection

- Joint aspiration is the removal of fluid from a joint, which then can be analysed in the laboratory and used for diagnosis. If a joint is very swollen, aspiration may also relieve the pressure in the joint and so reduce the pain.

- Aspiration is sometimes followed by an injection of a corticosteroid drug and local anaesthetic into the joint. The corticosteroid reduces inflammation, while the local anaesthetic relieves pain more quickly.

- The procedure is usually carried out in the out-patient clinic. Your doctor will make sure that your joint is in a comfortable position, and you should try to relax the joint and surrounding muscles

- A needle is inserted into the joint. For most joints this is very simple, and local anaesthetic is not needed beforehand. Joint fluid is drawn out through the needle and, if needed, corticosteroid and local anaesthetic are injected through the same needle.

- The injection site may be covered with a plaster, which can be removed after about a day. There is no harm in getting the area wet.

- Rest the joint as much as possible for a day after the injection. The discomfort may get slightly worse at first, and it may take a day or two before you feel a benefit. But, if the joint becomes very painful and swollen after the injection, contact your family doctor straight away.

The shoulder

- Tendon
- Capsule
- Bone
- Joint space
- Muscle

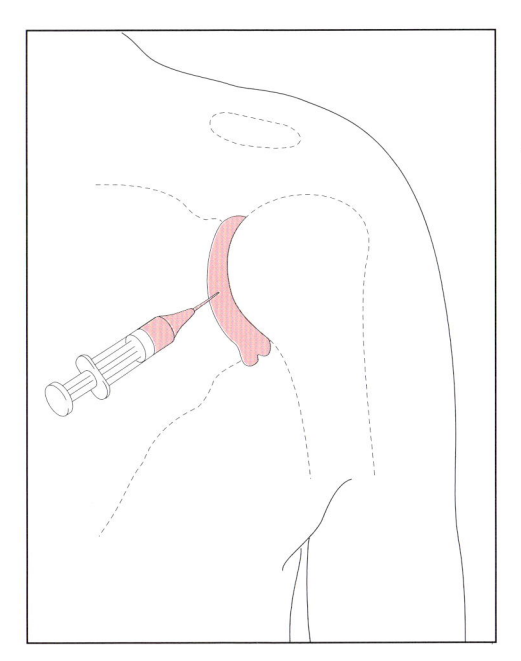

Aspiration and injection of the shoulder joint

© Health Press Limited

Soft tissue injections

- Inflammation of the soft tissues, which are the ligaments, tendons and bursae, often responds to treatment with a corticosteroid injection.

- A bursa (plural is bursae) is a pocket of fluid lying between the bone and skin, or bone and tendon. It prevents the bone from rubbing on, and damaging, nearby structures. The lining of the bursa is similar to the lining of a joint and it can become inflamed in the same way. An example is housemaid's knee, which is inflammation of the bursa between the kneecap and skin.

- The skin over the injection site is cleaned with antiseptic. The injection is usually into, or close to, the tender area.

- Other examples of soft tissue inflammation are tennis elbow and golfer's elbow, trochanteric bursitis, which causes pain in the hip, and plantar fasciitis, which causes pain in the sole of the foot.

- Tennis elbow and golfer's elbow are caused by inflammation at the sites where the forearm muscle tendons attach to bone.

- The trochanteric bursa lies over the bony part of the hip at the upper, outer thigh. Inflammation here causes trochanteric bursitis.

- The plantar fascia is the tough ligament tissue forming the sole of the foot. Plantar fasciitis is inflammation at the point where it attaches to the bone beneath the heel, and it causes pain when you walk.

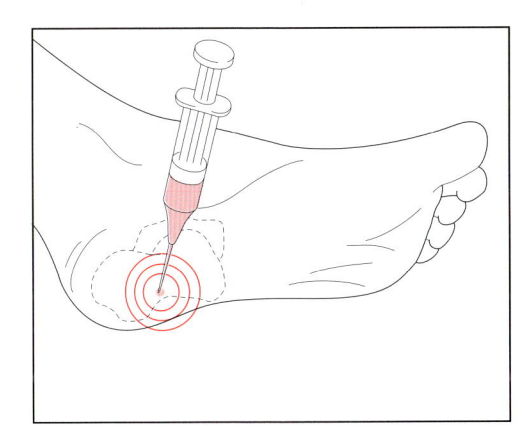

Injection for plantar fasciitis

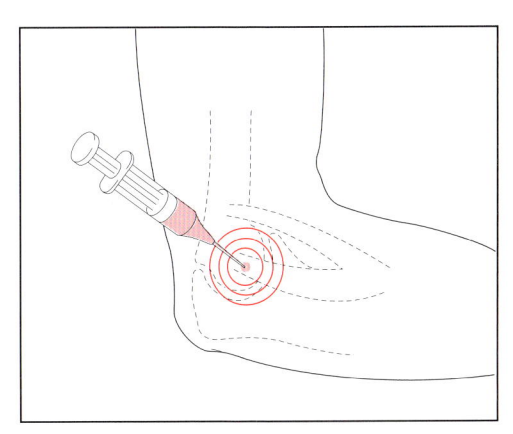

Injection for tennis elbow

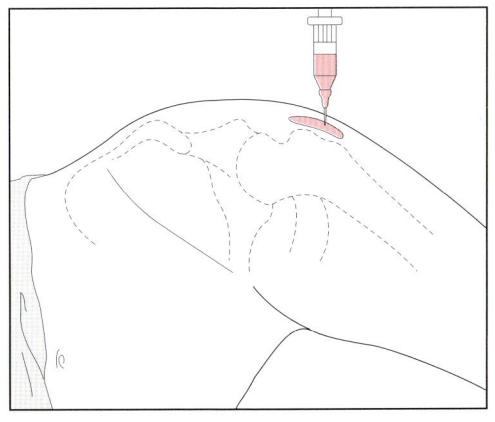

Injection for trochanteric bursitis

Carpal tunnel syndrome

- Carpal tunnel syndrome is caused by pressure at the wrist on one of the nerves supplying the hand. It occurs where the nerve passes under a tight band of fibrous tissue. There is often no underlying cause for this problem, though it may happen with rheumatoid arthritis. It is also common in pregnancy.

- Symptoms include tingling and numbness in the thumb and nearby fingers. Sometimes there is pain in the hand and arm, particularly at night. Your thumb may also feel weak.

- Treatment usually involves an injection of corticosteroid into the wrist.

- Sometimes a splint is prescribed to relieve pressure on the nerve.

- Occasionally, you may need an operation to relieve the pressure on the nerve.

10

Band of fibrous tissue

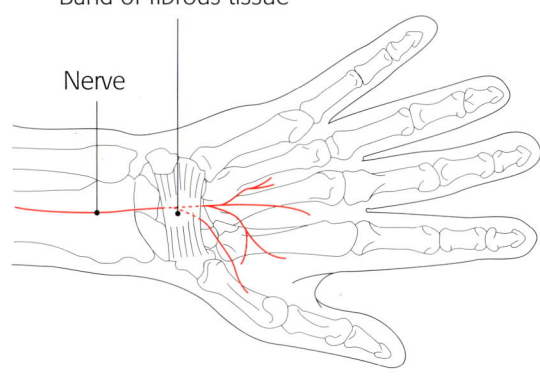

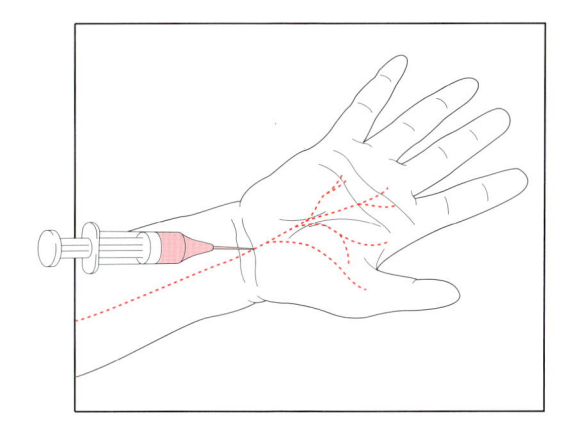

Nerve

Injection for carpal tunnel syndrome

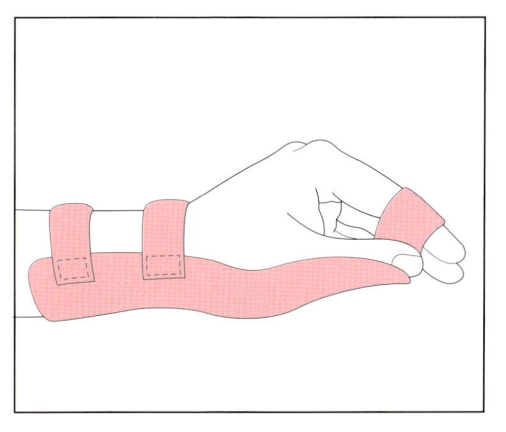

A splint for carpal tunnel syndrome

© Health Press Limited

Electromyography (EMG) and nerve conduction studies

- The electrical impulses produced by muscles and nerves are sometimes recorded to help diagnose damage to these structures.

- For muscle testing, a very fine needle is put into the muscle, and the muscle activity is recorded. This is called electromyography, or EMG for short. The results can show whether or not there is muscle damage.
  The procedure may cause minor twitching, but it is not painful.

- Nerve testing involves placing two probes on the skin, at points along the nerve. The nerve is stimulated with one probe, and a recording is made of the impulse reaching the other probe. This is called a nerve conduction study. Damage to the nerve is shown by changes in this impulse.

- For example, to diagnose carpal tunnel syndrome, the muscles at the base of the thumb may be tested. Also, the nerve supplying these muscles and the thumb and nearby fingers may be tested. The nerve will be stimulated on one side of the wrist, and a recording made on the other.

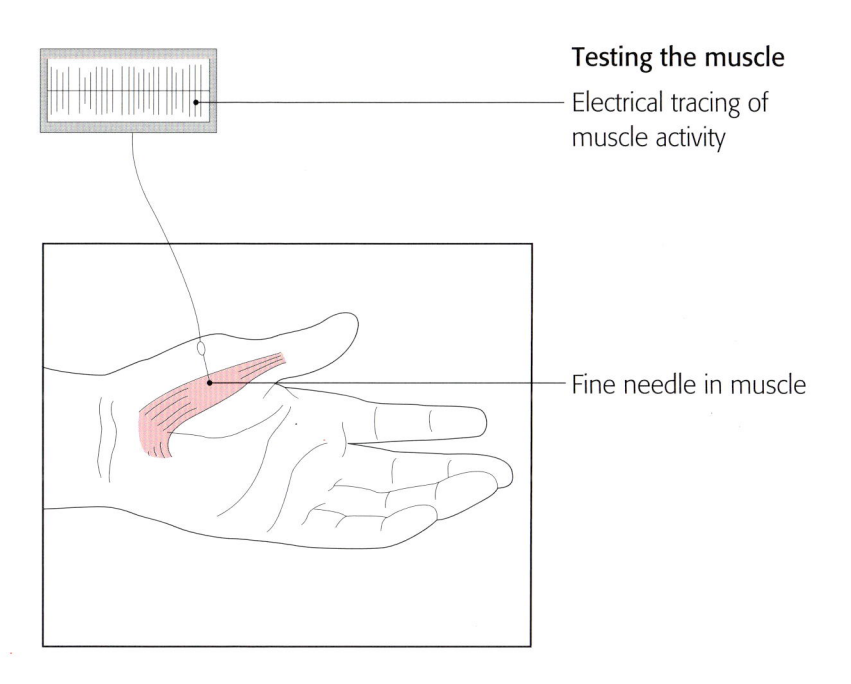

Testing the muscle

Electrical tracing of muscle activity

Fine needle in muscle

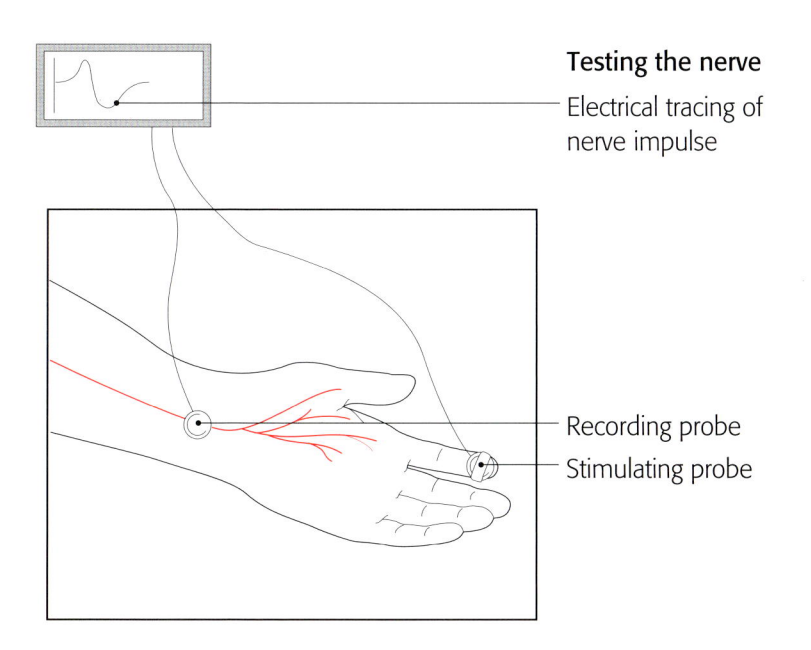

Testing the nerve

Electrical tracing of nerve impulse

Recording probe
Stimulating probe

Arthroscopy

- Arthroscopy allows the doctor to actually look inside the joint and may also be used for keyhole surgery. So, as well as helping diagnose joint disease, it may also form a part of the treatment.

- Arthroscopy is commonly performed on the knee, but can also be used for other joints, including those in the wrist and fingers.

- The procedure is carried out in an operating theatre under general or local anaesthetic.

- The arthroscope is a tiny telescope, which is inserted into the joint through a wider tube called a sheath. After the arthroscopy, there will be a small scar where the sheath passed through the skin. If you have surgery, it is carried out through a separate sheath, and there may be one or two other small scars if this has been done.

- After an arthroscopy, local anaesthetic and sometimes a corticosteroid drug are injected into the joint to reduce any pain. Often you can go home on the same day, but you may need to stay in hospital overnight.

- Rest your joint for 1 or 2 days after an arthroscopy. The doctor will probably place a thick pressure bandage over the joint which is usually removed 1 or 2 days later. If you have stitches, they will be removed after a few more days.

A normal knee

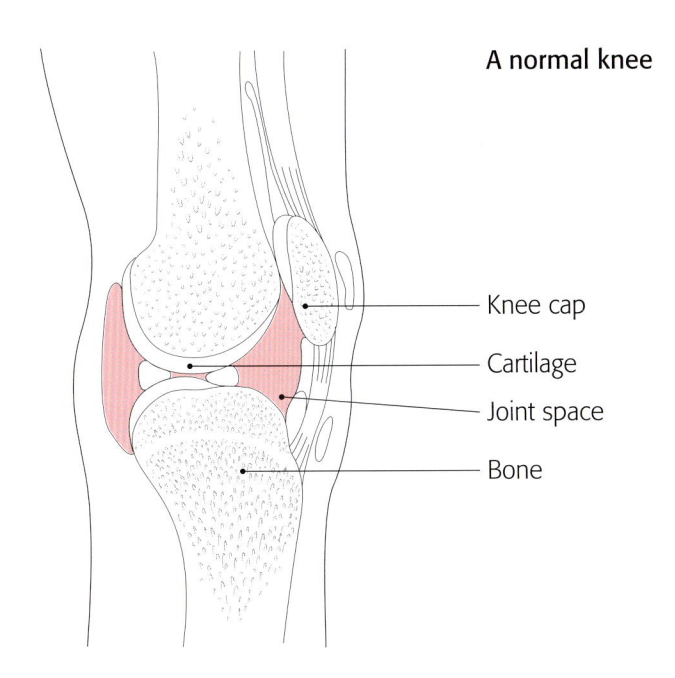

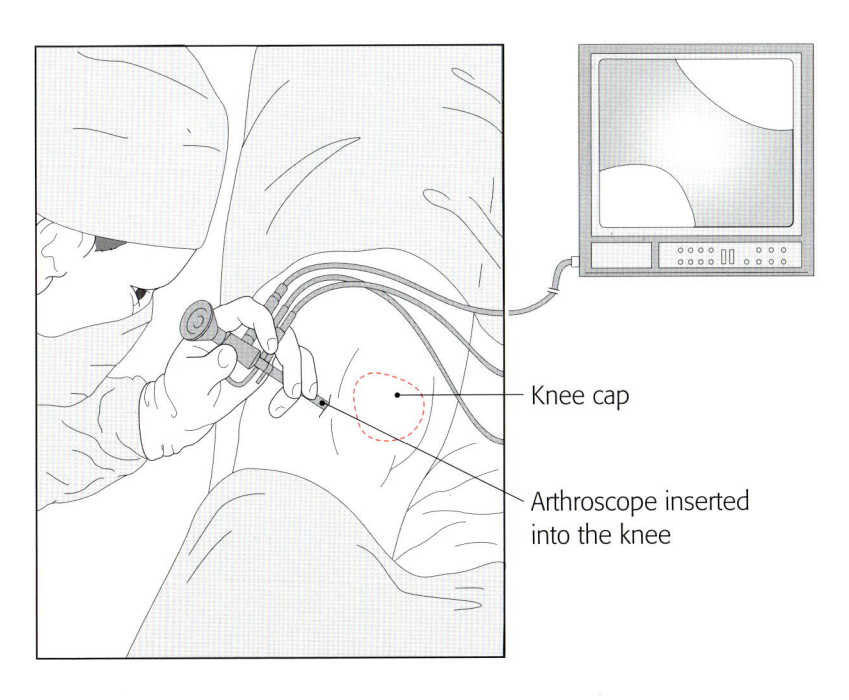

- Knee cap
- Cartilage
- Joint space
- Bone

- Knee cap
- Arthroscope inserted into the knee

Physiotherapy

- Physiotherapists are expert at helping joints and muscles recover from inflammation and damage.

- In general, you should rest an inflamed joint. But exercise is very important during the recovery phase, to prevent the surrounding muscles from wasting and becoming weak. Your physiotherapist will advise you on the best balance between exercise and rest.

- The physiotherapist can help with specific methods to reduce the inflammation and pain of arthritis. These include simple measures such as using ice packs to reduce swelling, or heat packs to ease pain. Other measures include ultrasound, and providing splints to ensure inflamed joints are rested in the proper position.

- Hydrotherapy involves exercising in a warm swimming pool. This allows joints to be exercised without stressing them too much.

- As joints recover, the physiotherapist will suggest graded exercises to gradually increase muscle strength.

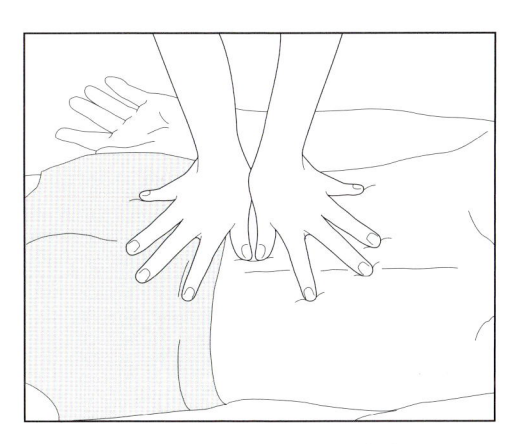

A mobilization technique for the lower spine

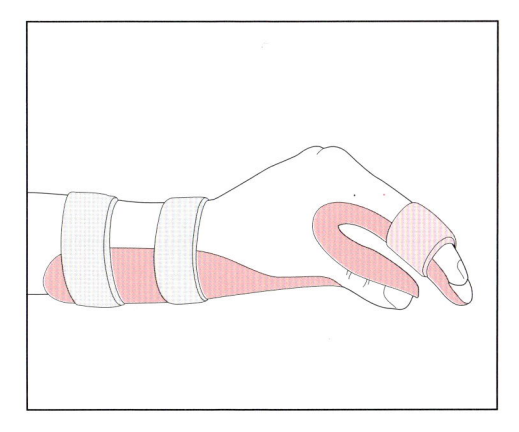

A 'resting' hand splint

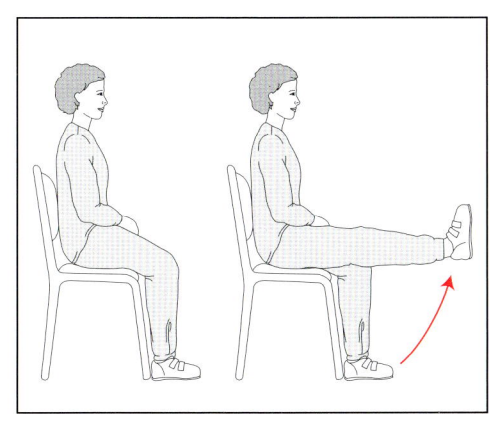

Simple exercises build up the muscles

Hydrotherapy

- Hydrotherapy involves exercise in a warm swimming pool.

- Warm water helps your muscles relax and your joints to move more. Water also supports the joints and reduces the stresses on them during exercise.

- Only short periods of time are spent in the pool, usually between 10 minutes and half an hour.

- It is important to have a drink afterwards and to rest, because hydrotherapy can be very tiring.

- It is usual to have a course of supervised hydrotherapy treatment. Afterwards you may be given advice on exercises to perform on your own in your local swimming pool.

- You do not need to be able to swim to attend hydrotherapy. If you cannot manage steps, there is usually a lift to help you into the pool.

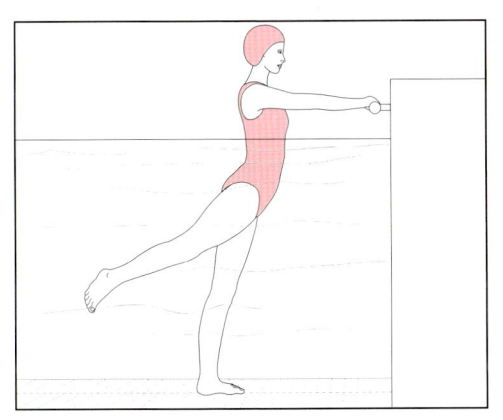

Exercises in the pool can be carried out in a variety of ways, including free-standing, using equipment or with the help of a physiotherapist

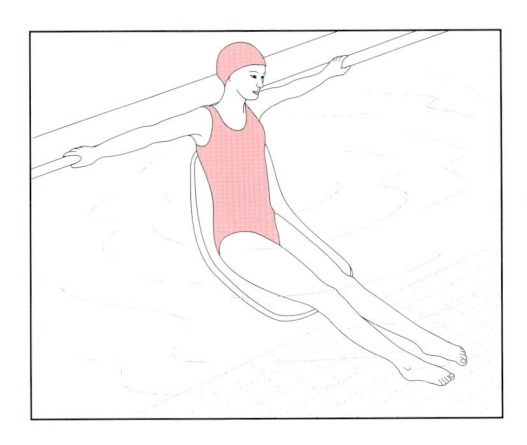

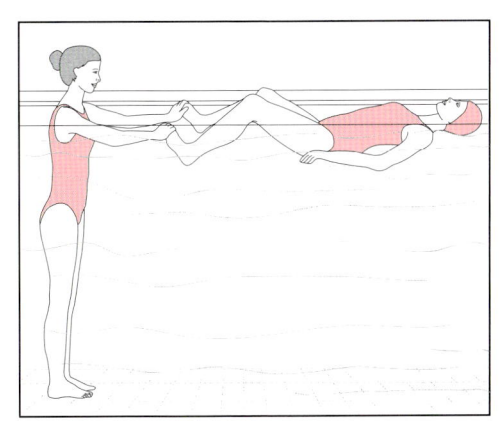

Occupational therapy

- Occupational therapists can show you how to protect your joints and can teach you how to live with inflamed and damaged joints without making the damage worse.

- They are also skilled in assessing how well your weakened or damaged joints can move. They can also provide help in making everyday life easier.

- The occupational therapist may supply gadgets to help you in the kitchen. For example, you may receive devices to help you open tins, or to hold a knife and fork more easily. Other gadgets may help you to pick up items without bending down.

- The occupational therapist may recommend changes to your home, such as a rail to help you get in and out of the bath, or higher chairs.

- Hand and wrist splints may be prescribed by the occupational therapist. 'Working' splints protect your hands and wrists during daily life, and spread the pressure evenly across damaged joints, so preventing further damage. 'Resting' splints are worn at night to prevent the development of deformities when your hands are resting.

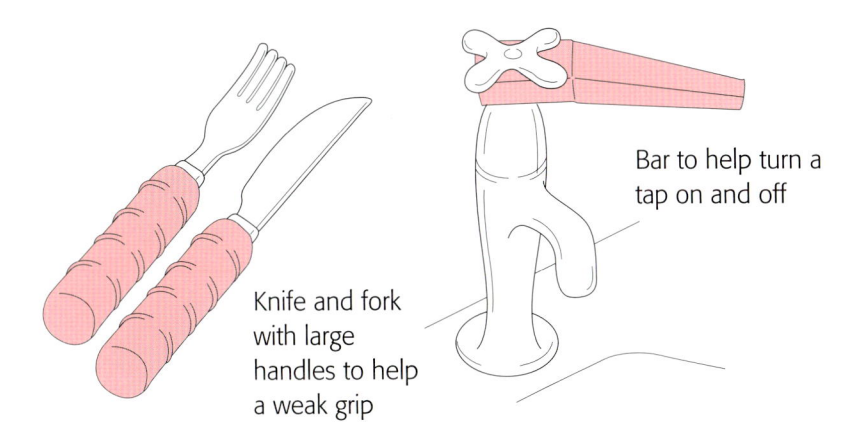

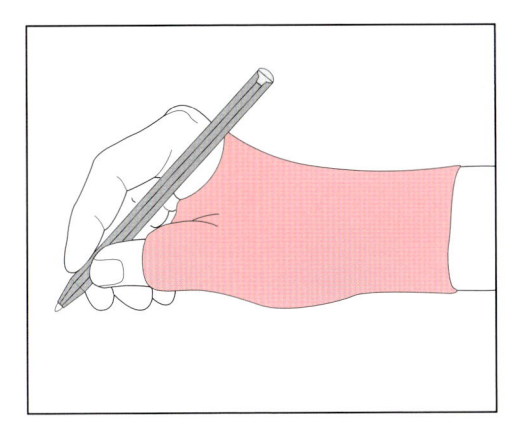

Knife and fork with large handles to help a weak grip

Bar to help turn a tap on and off

'Working' wrist splint

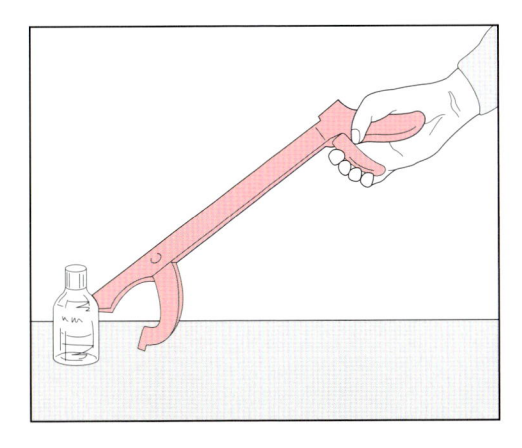

A 'helping hand'

The orthotist

- The orthotist is skilled in assessing deformities and stresses across joints.

- When joints become damaged, the physical stresses across the joints that occur as a result of daily living may increase the damage and deformity. This is particularly true for the joints of the foot and leg.

- As with the hands and wrists, splints can be used to reduce the damage. However, this is more difficult in the feet, and the orthotist may make adjustments to shoes or design inserts to wear inside the shoes instead.

- Occasionally you may need to have a pair of shoes 'made-to-measure'.

- The physiotherapist and orthotist may work together if you need other aids, such as neck collars.

- With modern technology and materials, 'surgical appliances' or 'made-to-measure' footwear can be designed to blend in with your clothes.

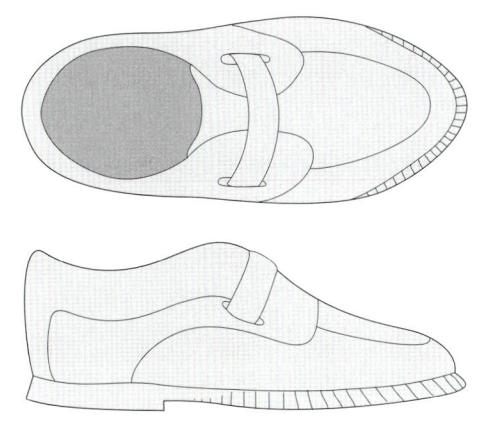

Made-to-measure shoes
They may be wide fitting, have velcro fasteners, or have inserts to support your feet

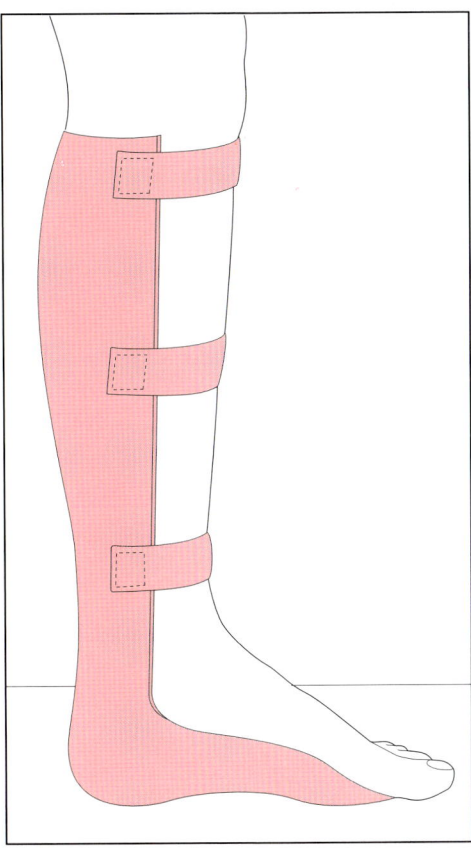

An ankle splint

The knee

- Pain in the knee can be caused by arthritis or by damage to the cartilage or ligaments in or around the joint. Damage can occur with all types of arthritis, but can also follow an injury, particularly from movements involving twisting. Inflammation can occur in the pocket of fluid lying in front of the knee. This pocket is called the pre-patellar bursa, and inflammation here causes housemaid's knee. Arthritis of the spine or hip can also sometimes cause knee pain. This is called referred pain.

- The events that occurred before the pain started, and the nature and exact location of the pain, will help the doctor decide what is causing it. Examination of the knee involves not only bending and straightening it, but also movements that stress the tendons and ligaments. Your back and hip may also be examined.

- Sometimes it may be necessary to drain fluid from the knee. This may be followed by an injection of corticosteroid drug and local anaesthetic. The corticosteroid reduces inflammation, while the local anaesthetic relieves pain more quickly.

- Your knee should be rested for a day after an injection. During this time, the discomfort may worsen slightly before it gets better. But, if the knee becomes very painful, and particularly if it becomes hot and swollen, you should contact your family doctor straight away.

- As the pain lessens, it is important to follow a regular exercise routine. You may be referred to a physiotherapist for advice on this.

Pre-patellar bursa

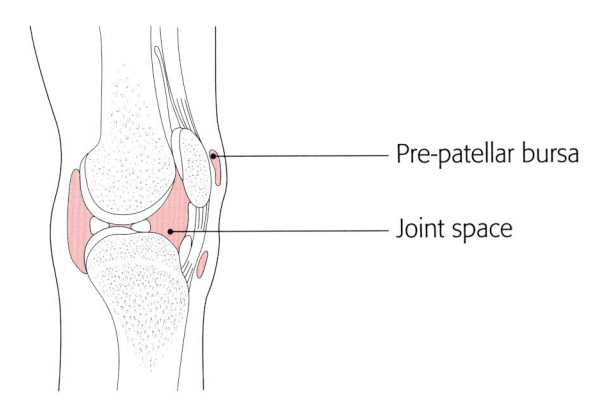

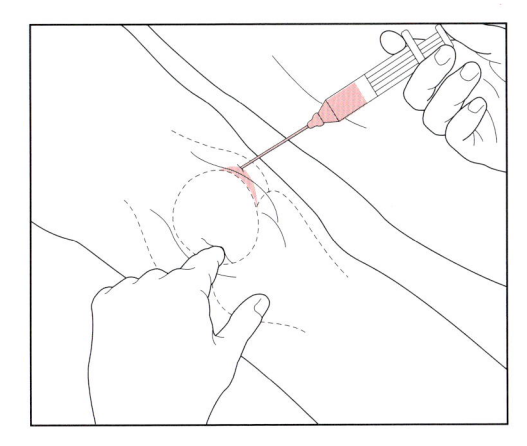

Joint space

Aspirating and injecting the knee joint

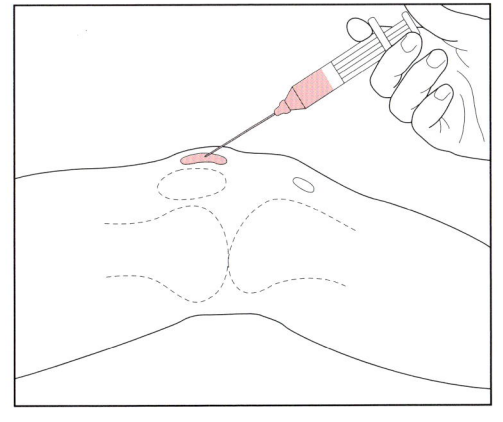

Aspirating and injecting the pre-patellar bursa

The shoulder

- The shoulder is our most complicated joint. Pain in the shoulder can come from the joint itself or the surrounding capsule, tendons or ligaments. Inflammation of the capsule eventually leads to a frozen shoulder, with very restricted movement.

- Shoulder pain is usually felt in the upper arm. It is usually impossible to sleep lying on the same side as the bad shoulder.

- Sometimes an injection may be needed to relieve the pain. The needle may be inserted either into the shoulder joint itself or into the pocket of fluid called the subacromial bursa, which lies above the joint. Depending on the origin of the pain, the front, back or side of the shoulder may be injected. The injection contains a corticosteroid drug and a local anaesthetic. The corticosteroid reduces inflammation, while the local anaesthetic relieves pain more quickly.

- Your shoulder should be rested for a day after an injection. During this time, the pain may worsen slightly before it gets better. But, if the shoulder becomes very painful, and particularly if it becomes hot and swollen, you should contact your family doctor straight away.

- As the pain lessens, it is important to follow a regular exercise routine. You may be referred to a physiotherapist for advice on this.

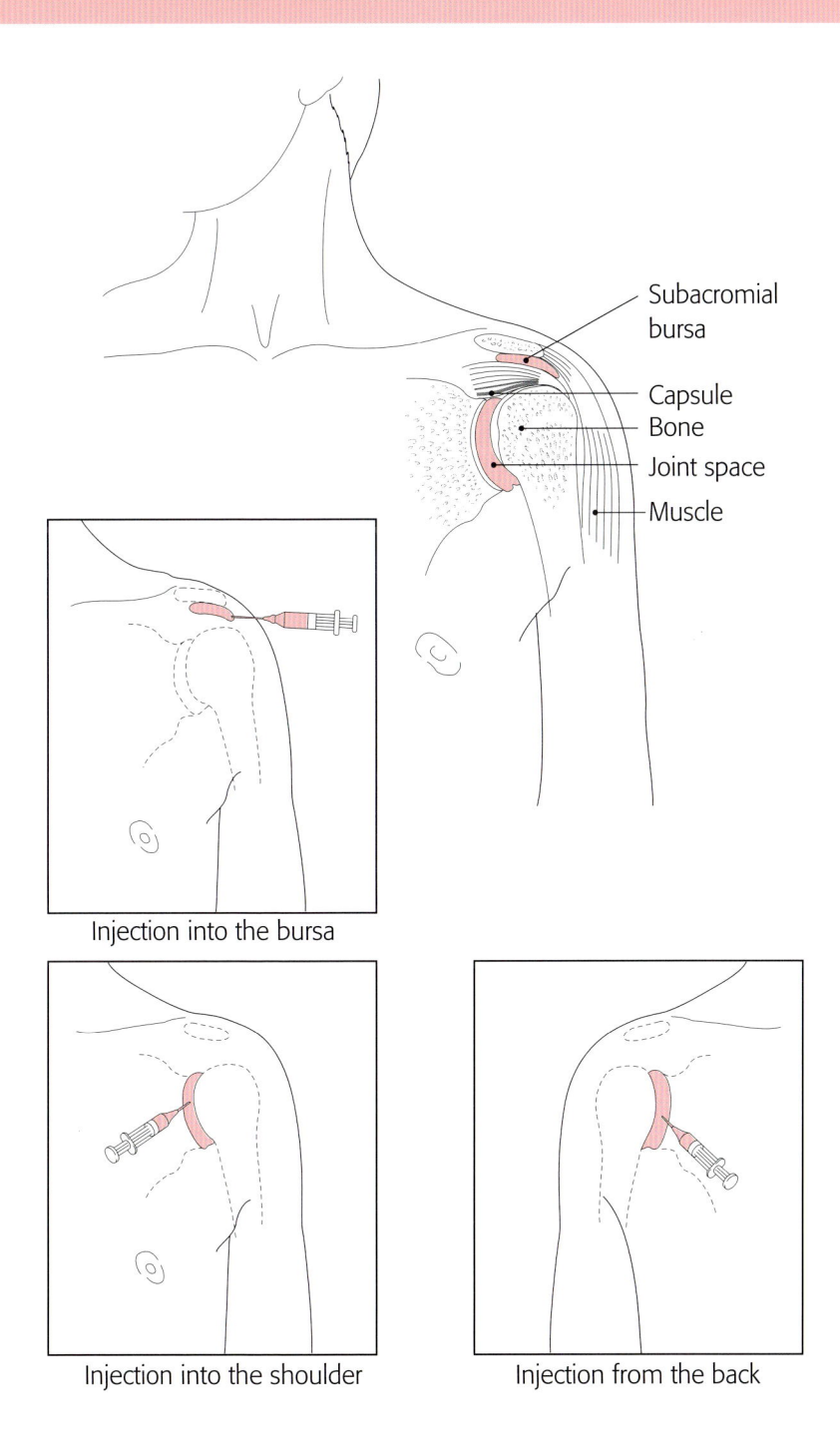

Subacromial bursa
Capsule
Bone
Joint space
Muscle

Injection into the bursa

Injection into the shoulder

Injection from the back

The wrist

- Pain in the wrist can come from the wrist joint itself or from inflammation of the tendons overlying the joint (tenosynovitis). Tenosynovitis may be caused by repetitive movements, but is also common in rheumatic illnesses.

- Sometimes it may be necessary to drain fluid from the wrist. This may be followed by an injection of corticosteroid drug and local anaesthetic. The corticosteroid reduces inflammation, while the local anaesthetic relieves pain more quickly.

- The needle is usually inserted into the top or side of the wrist.

- Your wrist should be rested for a day after an injection. During this time, the pain may worsen slightly before it gets better. But, if the wrist becomes very painful, and particularly if it becomes hot and swollen, you should contact your family doctor straight away.

- As the pain lessons, it is important to follow a regular exercise routine. You may be referred to a physiotherapist or occupational therapist for advice on this.

- Because the wrist is subjected to many stresses during daily use, you may need to wear a splint, especially when the wrist is inflamed. This spreads the pressure more evenly across the wrist and prevents further damage to the joint. The splint will be supplied by your physiotherapist or occupational therapist.

Joint space

Wrist joint

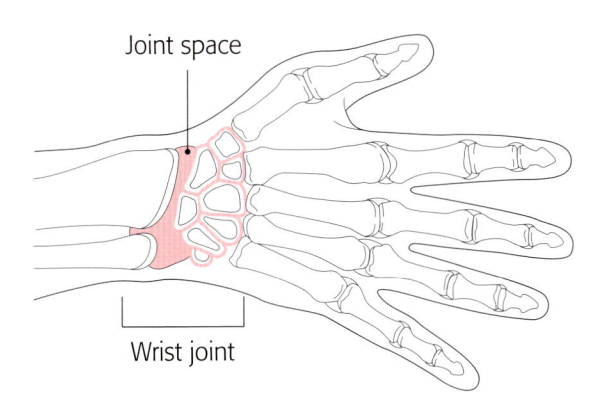

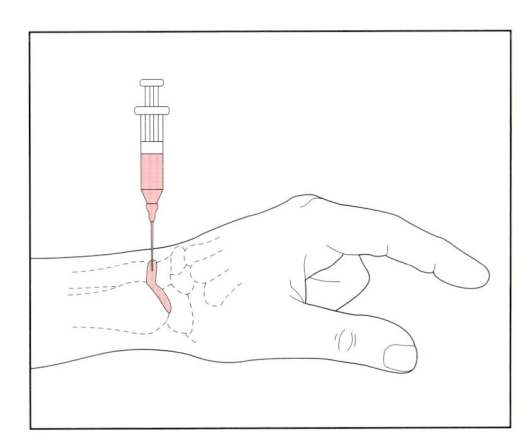

Injection into the wrist joint

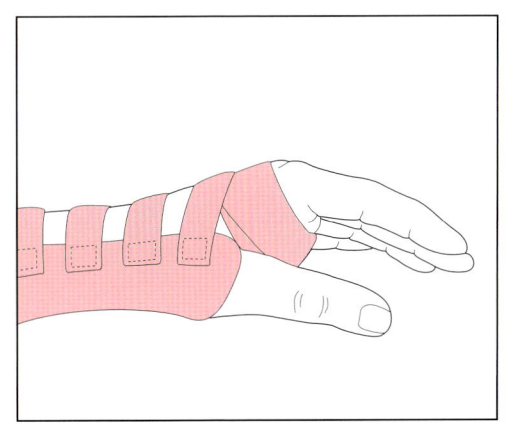

A wrist splint

The hand

- Pain in the hand may come from the joints of the hand and fingers or from inflammation of the tendons supplying the fingers, called tenosynovitis.

- Tenosynovitis may arise from repetitive movements, but it is also common in rheumatic illnesses. It may be associated with a 'trigger-finger', which is when you are able to bend a finger normally, but can only straighten it again by forcing it with the other hand.

- Sometimes it may be necessary to inject one or two joints, or the tendon sheaths, with a corticosteroid drug to reduce inflammation.

- The joint at the base of the thumb is injected through the side of the wrist. Tendon sheaths are usually injected through the palm of the hand at the base of the fingers.

- Your hand should be rested for a day after an injection. During this time, the pain may worsen slightly before it gets better. But, if the hand becomes very painful, and particularly if it becomes hot and swollen, you should contact your family doctor straight away.

- As the pain lessens, it is important to follow a regular exercise routine. You may be referred to a physiotherapist or occupational therapist for advice on this. You may also need to wear a splint during the day or at night.

20

Small joints of the fingers

Tendon sheath

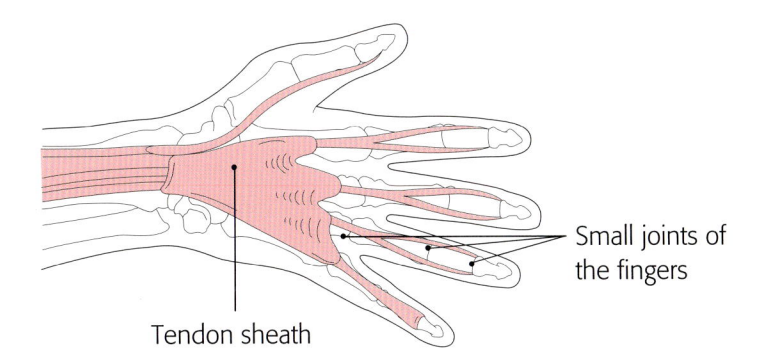

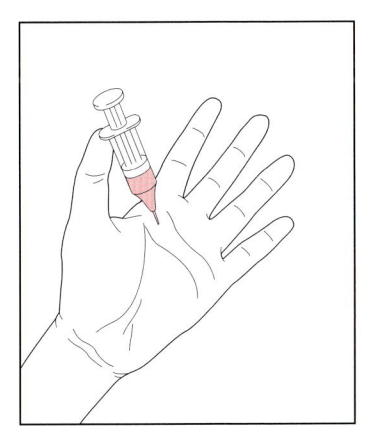

Injection into the tendon sheath

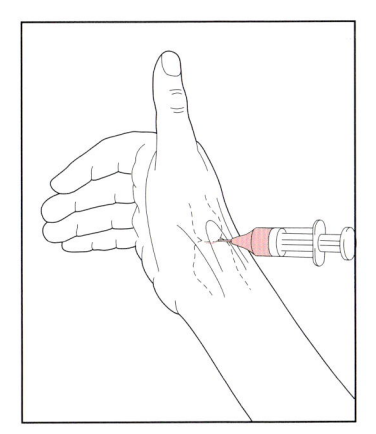

Injection into the joint at the base of the thumb

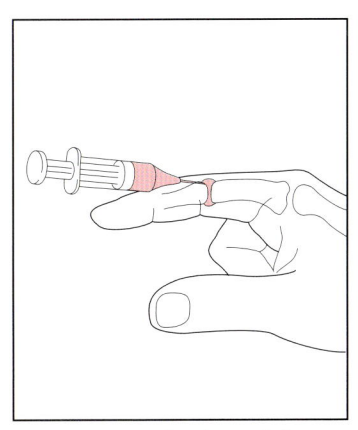

Injection of a finger joint

© Health Press Limited

The foot

- Foot pain can come from the joints of the foot, or from damage to the tendons or ligaments. Such damage may be caused by injury or inflammation. In arthritis, pain commonly arises from pressure on damaged joints or stretched ligaments during walking.

- Sometimes it may be necessary to inject one or two joints with a corticosteroid drug, to reduce inflammation. The needle is usually inserted into the side of the joint.

- Your foot should be rested for a day after an injection. During this time, the pain may worsen slightly before it gets better. But, if the foot becomes very painful after an injection, and particularly if it becomes hot and swollen, you should contact your family doctor straight away.

- As the pain lessens, it is important to exercise regularly; you may be referred to a physiotherapist for advice.

- Because the foot and ankle joints are subjected to higher stresses than any other joints during daily use, it is very important that they are protected properly. Modifications to shoes or inserts for shoes may be helpful. As well as relieving pain, these prevent too much pressure occurring across any particular joints that might increase the damage. In some situations, you may be referred to an orthotist to have shoes or splints 'made-to-measure'.

- Wearing trainers or using cushioned insoles reduces the impact of walking on hard ground. This can relieve pain and prevent further damage to the foot, knee, ankle or hip joints.

21

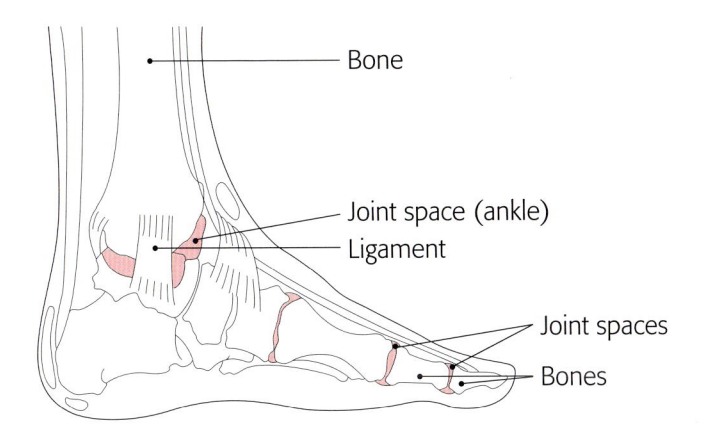

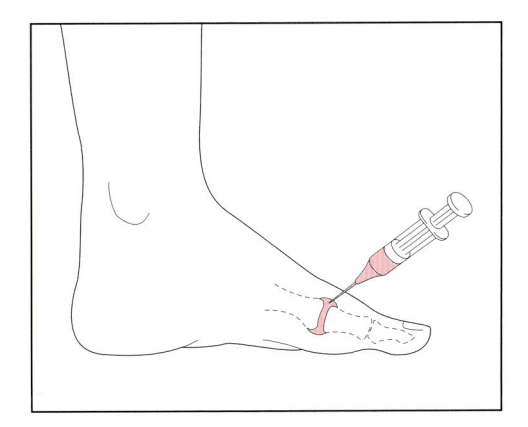

Bone

Joint space (ankle)
Ligament

Joint spaces
Bones

Injection of a joint of the foot

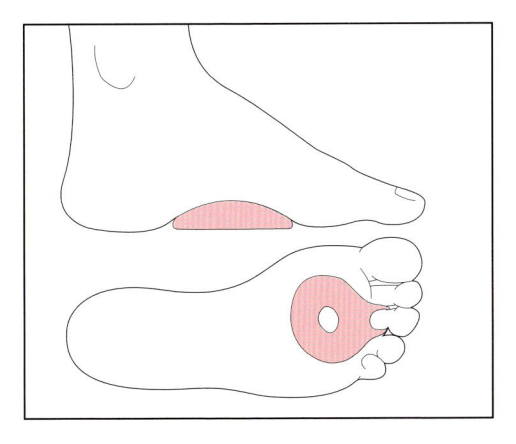

Arch support and metatarsal pad

The elbow

- Pain in the elbow can come from the elbow joint itself, or from inflammation of the tendons near to the joint, as in tennis elbow and golfer's elbow. Inflammation of the tendons may result from repetitive movements, but is also common in rheumatic illnesses. The pocket of fluid, called the bursa, lying over the point of the elbow may also become inflamed, and this condition is called olecranon bursitis.

- Sometimes it is necessary to drain fluid from the elbow, or to inject the elbow with a corticosteroid drug and a local anaesthetic. The corticosteroid reduces inflammation, while the anaesthetic relieves pain more quickly. With arthritis, the needle is usually inserted into the side or the back of the elbow.

- Your elbow should be rested for a day after an injection. During this time, the pain may worsen slightly before it gets better. But, if the elbow becomes very painful after an injection, and particularly if it becomes hot and swollen, you should contact your family doctor straight away.

- As the pain lessens after the injection, it is important to follow a regular exercise routine. You may be referred to a physiotherapist for advice on this.

- Tennis or golfer's elbow may be treated, at first, with rest and anti-inflammatory drugs. If these measures do not help, a corticosteroid drug may be injected into the tender area, to reduce inflammation.

Point of tenderness in tennis elbow

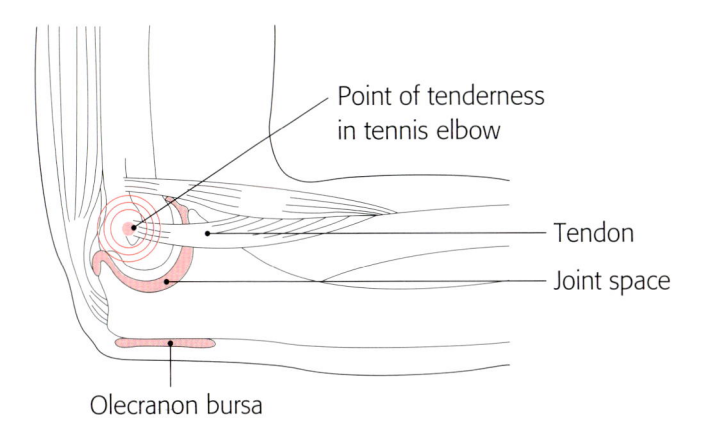

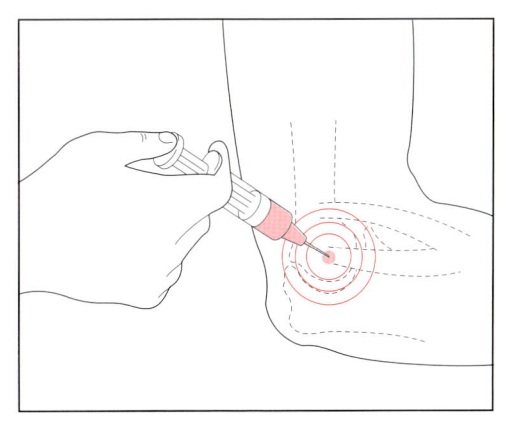

Tendon

Joint space

Olecranon bursa

Injection for tennis elbow

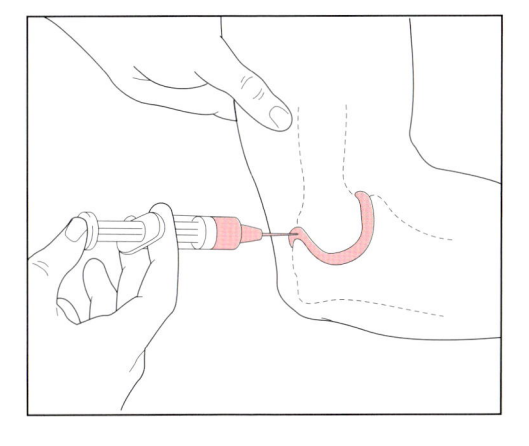

Injection into the elbow joint

The ankle

- Pain in the ankle may come from the ankle joint itself or from damage to the ligaments and tendons around the joint. Damage to the ligaments and tendons is usually the result of injury, particularly twisting movements. The Achilles tendon and nearby pockets of fluid, or bursae, may become inflamed in some rheumatic conditions.

- Sometimes it is necessary to drain fluid from the ankle, or to inject it with a corticosteroid drug and local anaesthetic. The corticosteroid reduces inflammation while the local anaesthetic relieves pain more quickly. Occasionally, it is necessary to inject the bursae next to the Achilles tendon.

- Your ankle should be rested for a day after an injection. During this time, the pain may worsen slightly before it gets better. But, if the ankle becomes very painful, and particularly if it becomes hot and swollen, contact your family doctor straight away.

- As the pain lessens, it is important to follow a regular exercise routine; you may be referred to a physiotherapist.

- If your ankle has been damaged by arthritis, there may be some deformity, and day-to-day walking can worsen it. Modifications to your shoes may be recommended to reduce pain and also to prevent further deformity.

- Wearing trainers or using special cushioned insoles reduces the impact of walking on hard ground. This can also prevent further damage to the joints in the foot, ankle, knee or hip.

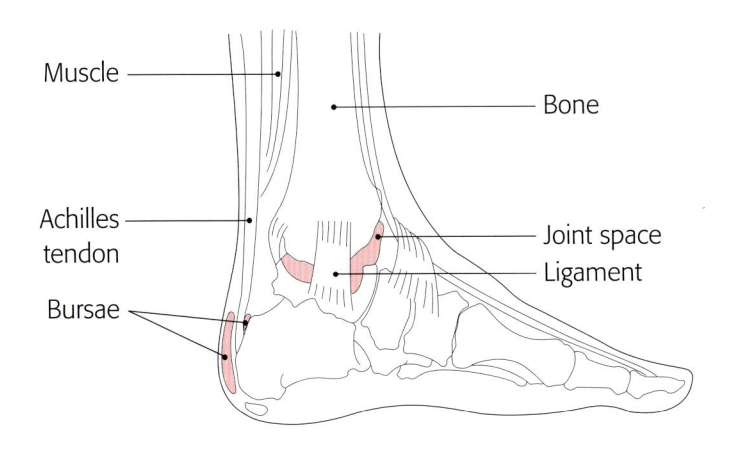

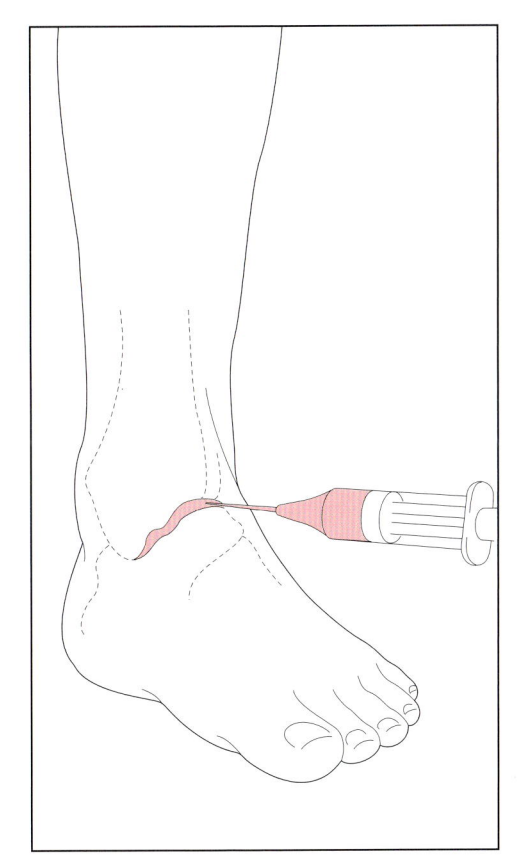

Muscle
Bone
Achilles tendon
Joint space
Ligament
Bursae

Injection into the ankle joint

The hips

- Hip pain is usually the result of 'wear-and-tear' arthritis, but the hips can sometimes be affected by inflammatory arthritis or infection. True hip pain is usually felt in the groin. Arthritis of the spine can also cause pain that appears to come from the hip, as can arthritis of the knee. This is called referred pain.

- Tronchanteric bursitis is inflammation of the pocket of fluid, or bursa, that lies over the bony part of the upper, outer thigh. It is a common condition that often occurs spontaneously, causing pain in the outside of the hip.

- Sometimes it is necessary to drain fluid from the hip, or to inject the hip with a corticosteroid drug and local anaesthetic. The corticosteroid reduces inflammation, while the local anaesthetic relieves pain more quickly.

- Unlike other joints, the hip joint is not easy to get to. Hip joints are therefore usually drained and injected in the X-ray department and the doctor uses X-rays or ultrasound to guide the needle into the joint. The needle is usually inserted into the groin for a hip injection.

- You should rest for a day after a hip injection. During this time, the pain may worsen slightly before it gets better. But, if the hip becomes very painful, you should contact your family doctor straight away.

- As the pain lessens, it is important to follow a regular exercise routine. You may be referred to a physiotherapist for advice on this.

24

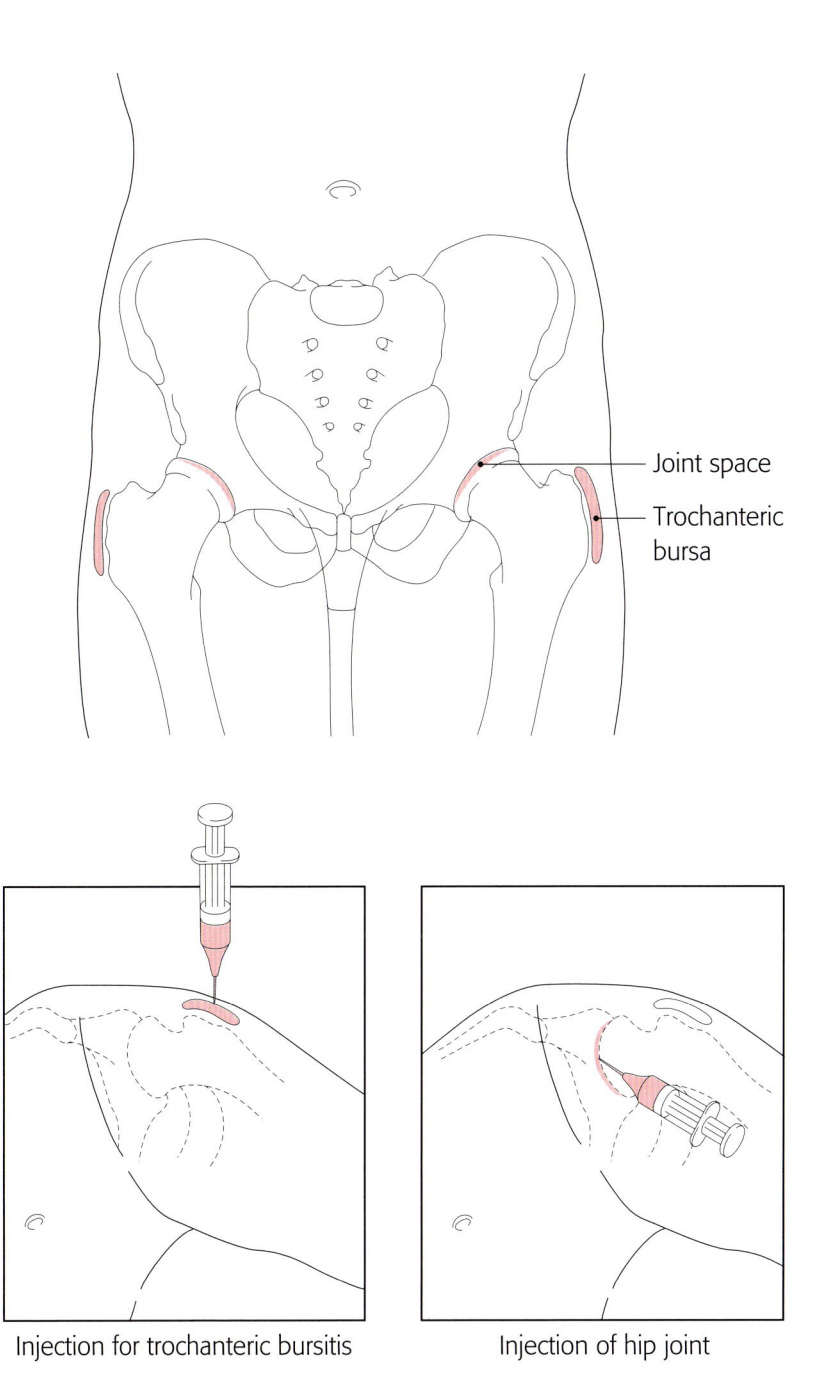

Joint space
Trochanteric bursa

Injection for trochanteric bursitis

Injection of hip joint

© Health Press Limited

The back

- Back pain, particularly lower back pain, is a major cause of ill-health. Lower back pain is often due to 'wear-and-tear' of the joints of the spine, in which case it is worse after activity, and made easier by rest.

- Less commonly, the spine and its ligaments can be affected by inflammation, known as spondylitis. This results in stiffness after periods of rest. It can affect the whole spine, as well as the sacro-iliac joints.

- In some cases, pain comes from the ligaments and muscles supporting the spinal bones. This is common with jobs that involve a lot of standing or sitting, particularly if your posture is poor. This is called back strain.

- As well as examining your back, the doctor may give you a thorough examination to rule out other causes of pain.

- Physiotherapy is very useful for back pain. The treatment depends on the problem, but may include exercises, traction, stretching of the back, hydrotherapy, heat and ultrasound. It helps correct abnormal posture, relieve muscle spasms and rebuild muscle strength. You may be encouraged to swim as this is an excellent form of exercise for back problems. Regular exercise is especially important for inflammatory back pain to prevent deformities developing.

- A firm bed and mattress may help to ease long-standing or regular back pain. Some patients find acupuncture or manipulation by an osteopath useful.

The bones and joints of the back

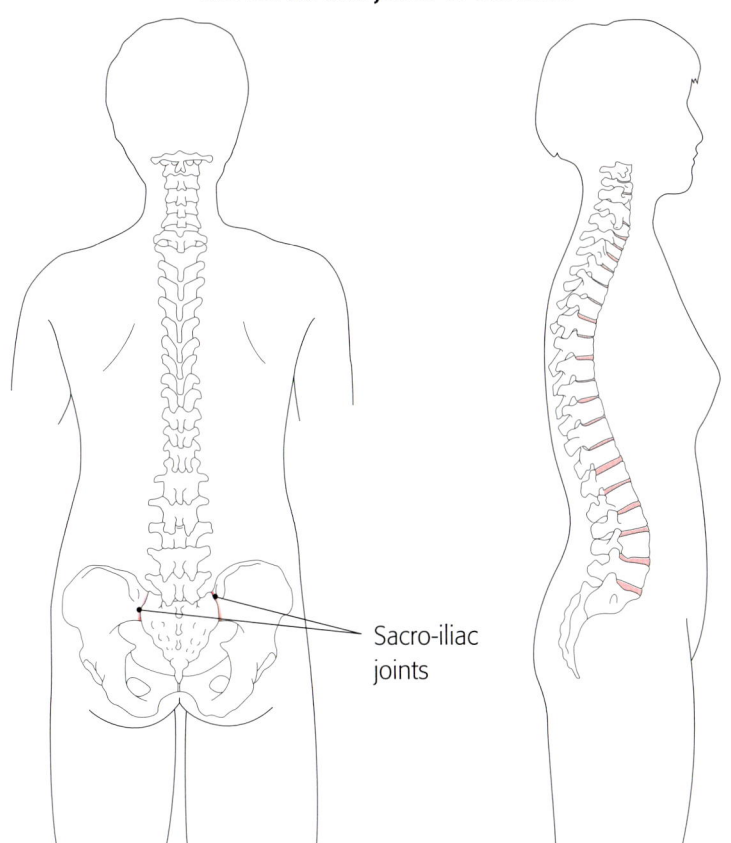

Sacro-iliac joints

Normal spine curvature

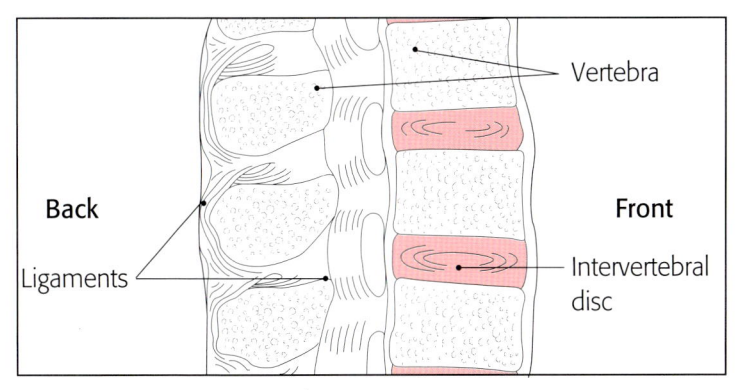

Vertebra

Back

Ligaments

Front

Intervertebral disc

Close up of the spine showing individual bones and joints

'Slipped' disc

- Discs are packets of fibrous tissue that separate the individual bones, or vertebrae, that make up the spine.

- Too much pressure or strain can cause a disc to 'give' and bulge out from between the vertebrae. This can result in pressure on nerves that run nearby, which causes pain in the areas of skin served by these nerves. Pain may be brought on by lifting heavy objects, but often there is no clear cause.

- Slipped discs usually occur in the low or lumbar spine, giving rise to pain in the back of the leg, or sciatica. Sometimes you may feel pain at the front or side of the leg. The pain is often brought on by coughing, sneezing or straining.

- As well as examining your back, the doctor will look for signs of nerve root irritation. This involves testing the sensation, power and reflexes in your legs. 'Straight leg raising', where the doctor lifts your leg while you lie on the couch, stretches the sciatic nerve, and may mimic your sciatic pain. The doctor may need to test the sensation of the skin around your back passage and genital area. Occasionally, your back passage will need to be examined internally.

- If the sciatic pain is severe, you may need to stay in bed for 1 or 2 days. However, you must get up and move around as soon as the pain eases.

- Physiotherapy can provide pain relief, as well as helping to get your back moving normally again.

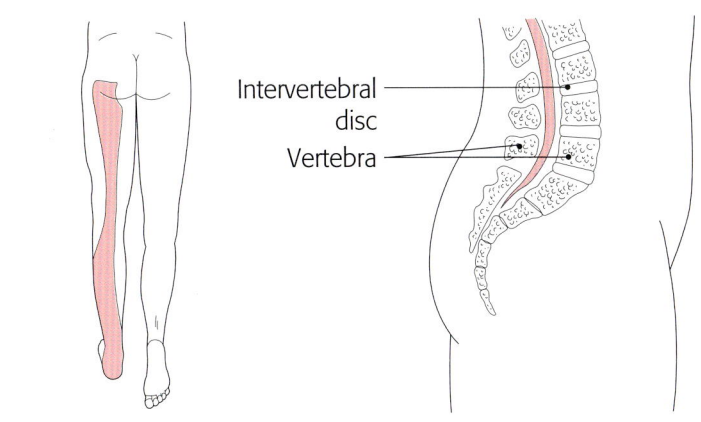

Common sites of sciatic pain

The lower lumbar spine
- Intervertebral disc
- Vertebra

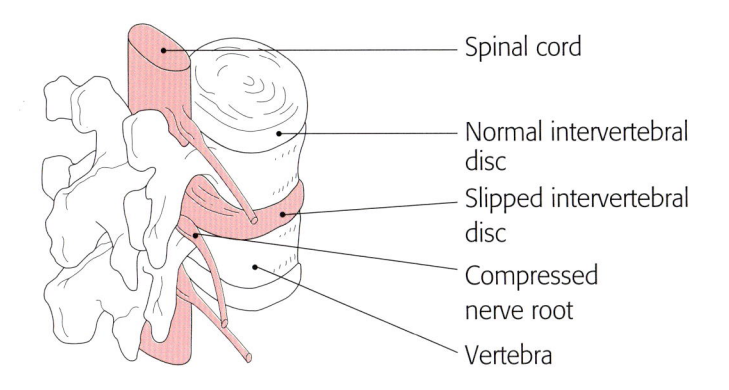

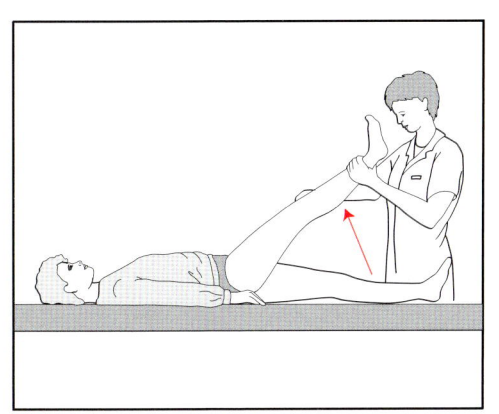

- Spinal cord
- Normal intervertebral disc
- Slipped intervertebral disc
- Compressed nerve root
- Vertebra

'Straight leg raising'

Ankylosing spondylitis

- Ankylosing spondylitis, or AS for short, causes back pain. With AS, the sacro-iliac joints and the small joints in the back become inflamed, which causes pain and stiffness, especially first thing in the morning. AS can also cause arthritis in other joints, such as the hips, knees and feet.

- Regular back exercises are very important for AS. They stop your spine becoming curved. Your physiotherapist will tell you what exercises to do and how often. They will also look at your posture and back movements from time to time to make sure that the exercises are working.

- Anti-inflammatory drugs help to reduce your symptoms. You may also be given so-called 'disease-modifying' drugs, particularly if you have arthritis in places other than the joints in your back.

- Occasionally, if your pain is severe, your doctor may inject local anaesthetic and a corticosteroid drug into your sacro-iliac joints. The corticosteroid helps to relieve the inflammation and the local anaesthetic relieves the pain more quickly.

- You should rest for a day after an injection. During this time the pain may worsen before it gets better. If your back becomes very painful, you should contact your doctor straight away.

- Some people with AS get inflammation in other parts of the body, especially the eye. This is called iritis, and it causes a painful red eye. It is treated with corticosteroid eye drops.

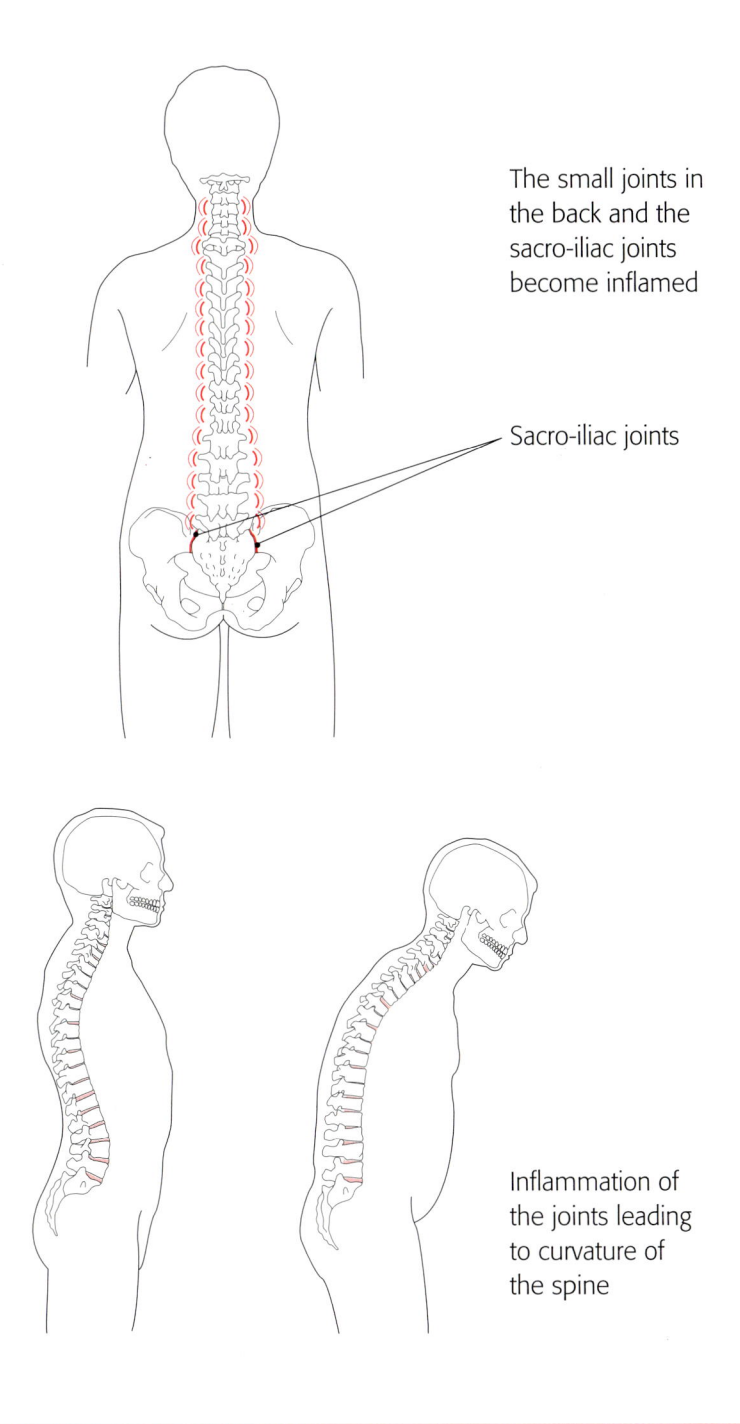

The small joints in the back and the sacro-iliac joints become inflamed

Sacro-iliac joints

Inflammation of the joints leading to curvature of the spine

Neck pain

- Neck pain is very common. It is usually the result of 'wear-and-tear' arthritis, but can also occur with rheumatoid arthritis. It may simply be caused by poor posture.

- Occasionally, arthritis in the neck can result in 'trapped nerves' and this can cause tingling, pain and weakness in your shoulders, arms and hands, or headaches. Rarely, neck arthritis can cause damage to the spinal cord, which may cause weakness in the legs.

- The rheumatologist will assess your neck movements, and examine your arms and legs. An X-ray may be taken.

- A combination of rest and physiotherapy relieves most cases of neck pain. Physiotherapists can use heat and ultrasound to reduce inflammation in the neck, and can also help tense and stiff muscles to relax. Traction or stretching of the neck can be helpful when there are symptoms from trapped nerves.

- You may need to wear a collar for a short while to rest the neck. It is also important to make sure your work is not causing problems. For example, computer monitors must be at an appropriate level to prevent abnormal neck postures and your chair should support your back properly.

- Most neck problems recover with treatment. If your symptoms return look for causes, particularly at work.

The neck

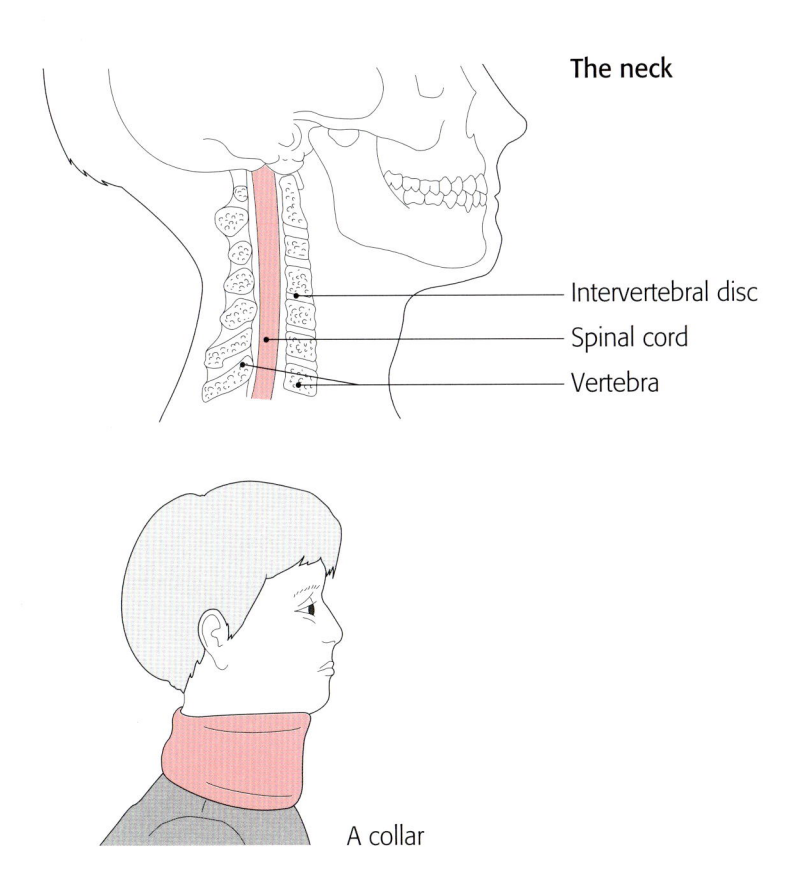

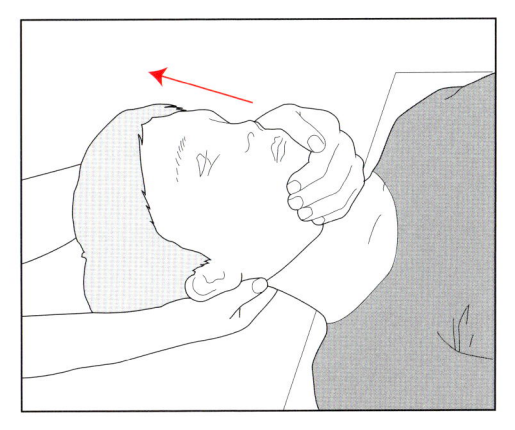

- Intervertebral disc
- Spinal cord
- Vertebra

A collar

Traction

Osteoporosis

- Osteoporosis, or thin bones, most commonly affects women after the menopause. This is when the level of the female sex hormone called oestrogen falls, and it is this hormone that keeps the bones strong.

- There are other risk factors for osteoporosis, such as heavy smoking or drinking, long-term treatment with corticosteroid drugs, and surgical removal of the ovaries before the menopause. Rheumatoid arthritis can cause osteoporosis, and the condition can also run in families.

- There are many consequences of osteoporosis. You may develop severe back pain because the vertebrae of the spine eventually collapse and become flattened. You may lose height and develop a stoop. You are also more likely to break your bones, particularly your hip and wrist.

- X-rays or CT scans may be used to determine your bone strength but, where available, you will have a formal 'bone density' measurement. This is similar to having standard X-rays taken of your back and hip.

- Osteoporosis is commonly treated with hormone replacement therapy (HRT). There are various forms of HRT, and not all of them cause your periods to start again. Other forms of treatment include calcium and vitamin D supplements, and drugs called bisphosphonates. Regular exercise and a healthy diet are very important.

Common places where bones break with osteoporosis

- Spine
- Hip
- Wrist

Normal spine

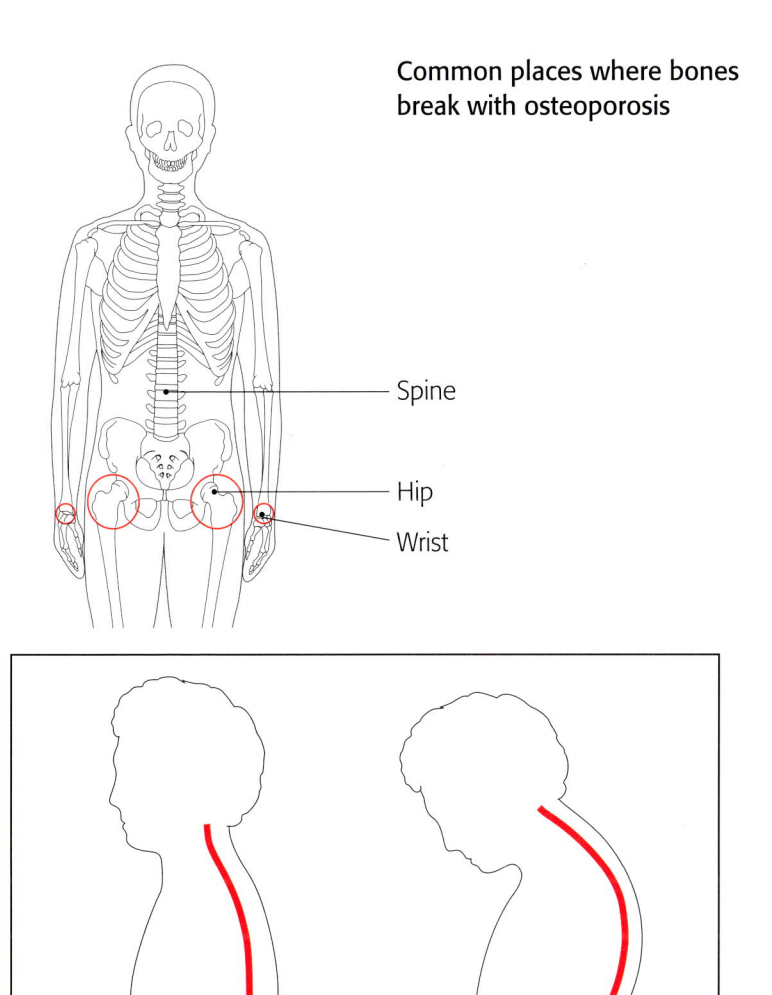

Osteoporotic spine

Normal vertebrae

'Crushed' vertebrae

Sjögren's syndrome

- Sjögren's syndrome can occur on its own, or with other rheumatic conditions. It causes dry eyes and mouth because the glands that produce tears and saliva become inflamed and dry up.

- Your eyes may feel gritty and sticky, especially first thing in the morning. A dry mouth makes you feel thirsty all the time.

- To diagnose the condition, your doctor may place a small strip of blotting paper just inside your lower eyelid for a couple of minutes. This is not painful and measures your tear production.

- Another test is called a lip biopsy. This involves removing a tiny piece of tissue from your lip. It is a simple procedure performed by a surgeon, and is carried out under local anaesthetic.

- You may be given drops to soothe your eyes, and you may be advised to take regular sips of water. You may also be given an artificial saliva spray for your mouth.

- Sometimes an eye surgeon will block off your tear ducts, so that tears stay in your eyes for longer. It is a simple operation which only takes a few minutes, and is done under local anaesthetic.

- Sjögren's syndrome can also affect other glands in the body. Tell your doctor about any other symptoms as these can usually be treated. For example, the glands that produce vaginal fluid may dry up, making sex painful.

30

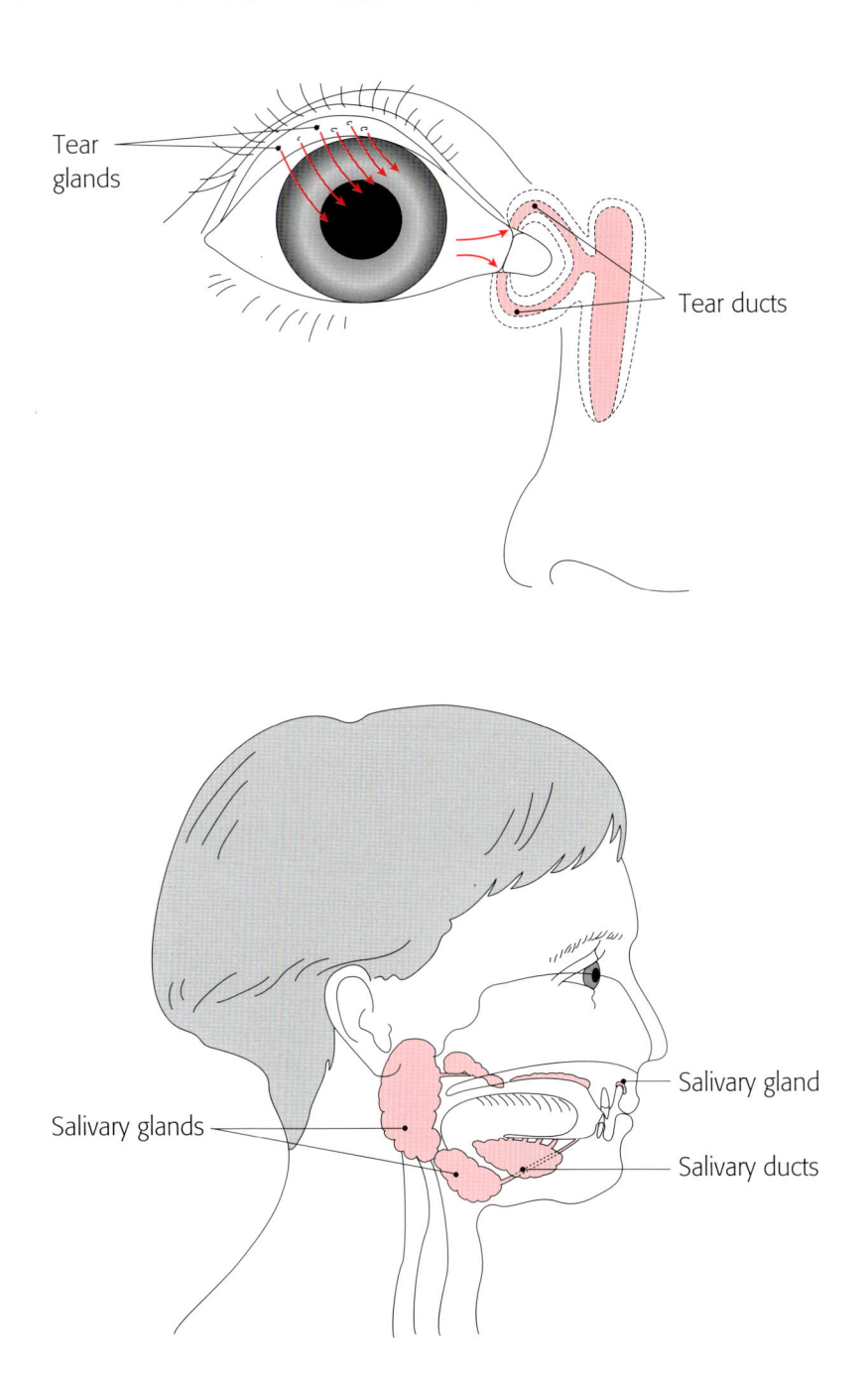

Hypermobility syndrome

- Your ligaments and tendons control exactly how much your joints can move.

- Some people have 'loose' tendons and ligaments and their joints can move more than other people's. At school, these people are often called 'double-jointed', though the technical name is hypermobility syndrome.

- Most people with hypermobility syndrome are completely healthy, and some make the most of it by becoming gymnasts or ballet dancers.

- A few people with hypermobility syndrome develop symptoms such as pain and aching after exercise. These symptoms may be caused by stretching of the tissues around their joints, when the joints move more than they should.

- Hypermobility syndrome is diagnosed by measuring the amount of movement in the hands, elbows, knees and hips.

- If you have hypermobility syndrome, a physiotherapist can advise you how to look after your joints. This involves regular exercise to strengthen the tendons and the tissue around the joints.

- It is important to understand that exercise is good for your joints as long as you don't overstretch them.

Hypermobility syndrome

Overstretching at the hip

Overstretching at the knees

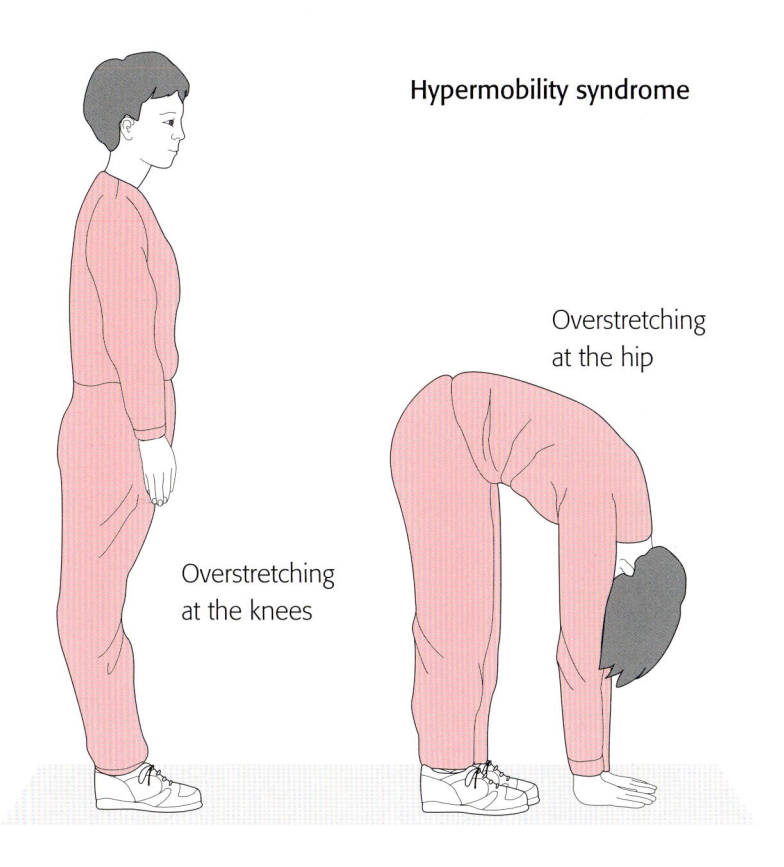

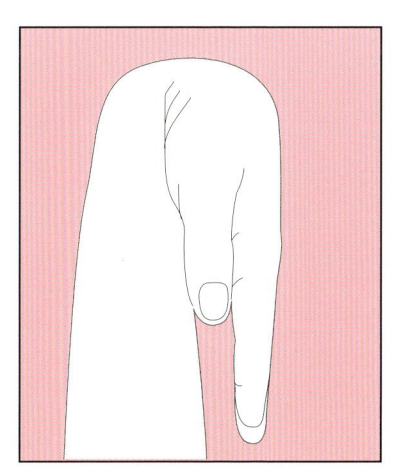

Overstretching the hand

Polymyalgia rheumatica

- Polymyalgia rheumatica, or PMR for short, is a common condition in the middle-aged and elderly. It causes severe pain and stiffness of the shoulder, neck and hip muscles and this is particularly bad first thing in the morning. It may be difficult to lift off the bedclothes or get out of bed, and you may feel generally unwell.

- Sometimes PMR is associated with inflammation of the arteries in the head and scalp, called temporal arteritis. This causes headaches, scalp tenderness, visual disturbances, and pain in the jaw muscles when eating.

- Diagnosis may not be easy, but a blood test called an ESR may show a very high reading. In the case of temporal arteritis, the doctor may take a tiny piece of tissue from one of the arteries running across your forehead. This is called a biopsy, and is performed in the operating theatre under general or local anaesthetic.

- PMR and temporal arteritis are usually treated with a corticosteroid drug, which gives rapid relief in a few days. You will need to continue treatment for up to 2 years, but the amount is gradually reduced so that you will only be taking a small dose after the first few months.

- Sometimes the disease 'flares up' as the corticosteroid dose is reduced, requiring a temporary increase. While taking corticosteroids, you should always carry a 'steroid card' which gives information about your medication. You should never stop taking corticosteroids suddenly.

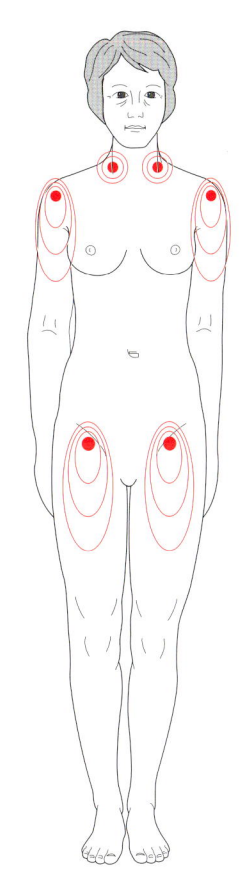

Areas of stiffness in polymyalgia rheumatica

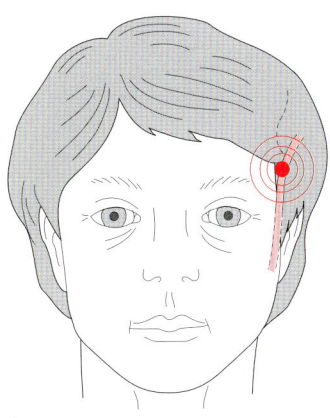

Area of headache and tenderness in temporal arteritis

Fibromyalgia

- Fibromyalgia, sometimes called fibrositis, is a common condition, particularly in middle-aged women. It causes muscle and joint aches and pains, which may be associated with severe tiredness and sometimes depression. You may have problems sleeping and feel exhausted when you wake up. The cause is unknown, but it is not life-threatening. Fibromyalgia is a real condition, and not something that is 'in the mind'.

- Diagnosis is difficult because there are no special features. All blood tests are normal, but you may be particularly tender in a few places, called 'trigger points'.

- There is some evidence that a poor sleep pattern in this condition leads to a vicious circle of poor sleep, resulting in more aches and pains, worse sleep, and so on. Your doctor may prescribe a small dose of antidepressant to take at night. You are not taking this for its antidepressant properties, but because it can correct your sleep pattern and help to relieve your symptoms.

- As your sleep pattern improves, you will be given a set of graded exercises to get back your muscle tone and power.

- With exercise and improved sleeping, the symptoms of fibromyalgia should ease over several months, although it may take longer. You may feel that exercise makes your symptoms worse, especially when you first start treatment. This is normal, and is not a sign that you are 'overdoing it'.

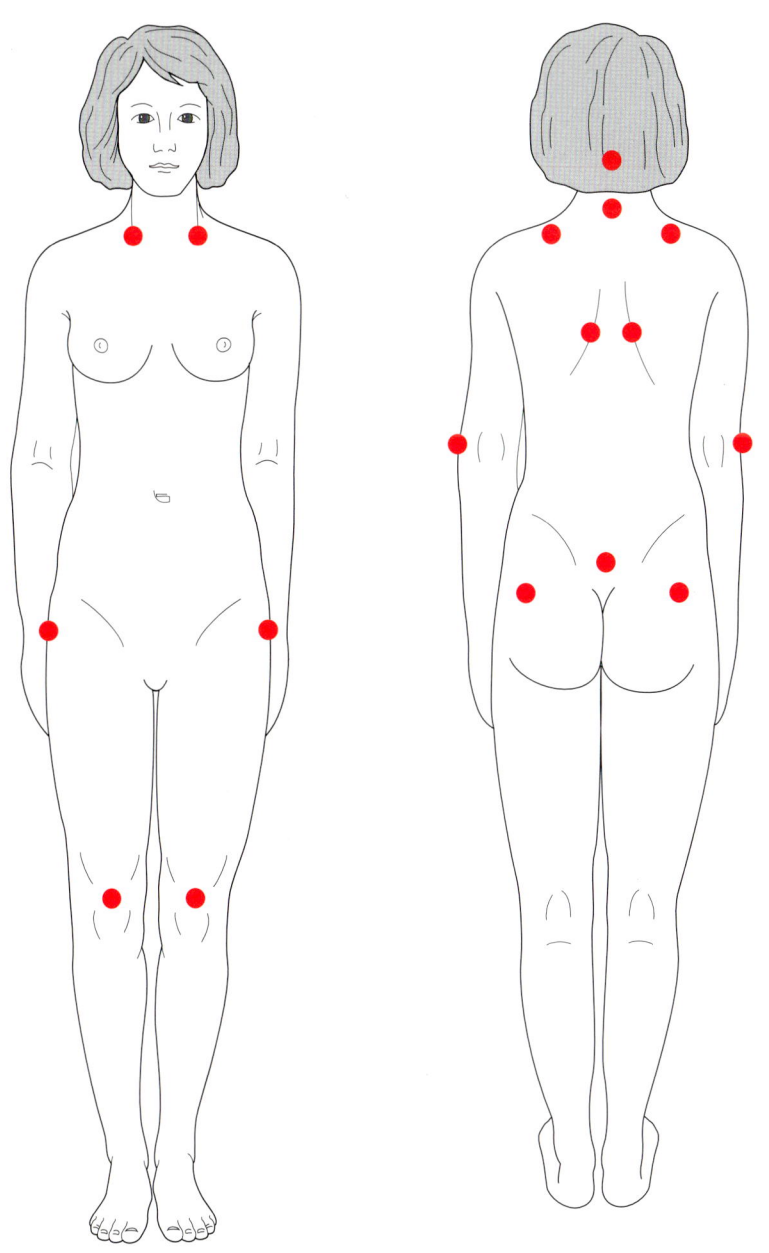

Tender sites in fibromyalgia

Mail Order

Visit our website at: www.patientpictures.com

This book is one of a rapidly growing series.

Current *Patient Pictures* titles:
- *Bladder disorders*
- *Cardiology*
- *End-stage renal failure*
- *Erectile dysfunction*
- *Fertility*
- *Gastroenterology*
- *Gynaecological oncology*
- *Gynaecology (2nd edition)*
- *HIV medicine*
- *Ophthalmology*
- *Prostatic diseases and their treatments*
- *Respiratory diseases*
- *Rheumatology (2nd edition)*
- *Urological surgery*

Forthcoming *Patient Pictures* titles:
- *Breast cancer*
- *ENT*

Call **1-800-538-1287** to order direct from the publisher, using your credit card

For an order form or an up-to-date list of *Health Press* titles, simply phone or fax:
Phone +44 1235 523233
Fax +44 1235 523238